Reiki
Best Practices

D1043439

Walter Lübeck
Frank Arjava Petter

Reiki
Best Practices

Wonderful Tools of Healing for
the First, Second, and Third Reiki Degree

Translated by Christine M. Grimm

LOTUS PRESS
SHANGRI-LA

Important Note: *Reiki—Best Practices* does not make the visit to a doctor, naturo-
path, or psychotherapist superfluous when there is a suspicion of a serious health
disorder. The information in this book has been portrayed to the best of our
knowledge and conscience. Despite this fact, the authors and the publisher will
not assume any type of liability for damages of any type that may occur from the
correct or incorrect use of the methods presented in this book. These are intended
as general information and for educational purposes.

The following term is a worldwide copyright by Walter Lübeck:
Rainbow Reiki KarmaClearing

Second Printing 2004
First English Edition 2003
©by Lotus Press
Box 325, Twin Lakes, WI 53181, USA
website: www.lotuspress.com
email: lotuspress@lotuspress.com
The Shangri-La Series is published in cooperation
with Schneelöwe Verlagsberatung, Federal Republic of Germany
© 2002 by Windpferd Verlagsgesellschaft mbH, Aitrang, Germany
All rights reserved
Translated by Christine M. Grimm
Edited by Neehar Douglass
Cover design by Peter Krafft, Design, Bad Krozingen, Germany,
using an illustration by Berthold Rodd
Illustrations: Martina Morlok: The drawings depict Frank Arjava Petter, Walter
Lübeck, and Veronika C. Wolfarth; Lisa Thiel was the model for the drawings on
pages 148 and 254

ISBN 0-914955-74-8

Library of Congress Control Number: 2003103525
Printed in USA

Table of Contents

---

* The capitals in brackets, WL for Walter Lübeck and FAP for Frank Arjava Petter show the author of the respective Reiki technique.

Preface

This book presents an overview of the Reiki treatment techniques that have been developed in the Western world. In it Frank Arjava and I endeavor to describe and explain particularly effective and useful 'Reiki tools'. Of course this collection is not and could not be definitive.

In recent decades many millions of Reiki enthusiasts throughout the world have developed so many wonderful ways to apply Reiki. These encompass such a vast spectrum of creativity that a work the size of the Encyclopedia Britannica would probably be necessary to portray all of them comprehensively.

In this book we seek to compile the Reiki techniques that are the most effective or are especially applicable for everyday use. We are looking to provide a detailed explanation of both their theory and their practice. This will allow you to find appropriate information and be inspired to develop your own techniques. At the same time you will learn a great deal about energy work with Reiki and spiritual healing in general.

Much of this material is being published for the first time or is being presented in detail not seen before. Some of the methods are described in different ways because Frank Arjava and I arise from different Reiki schools. We have maintained these differences to show that there are many paths leading to Rome and that it is for each of us to choose our own. We both fare well with this approach and hope, dear reader, that it will bring much good into your life also.

The time has come for all of us to work together to recreate paradise here on our planet. With this book we seek to show that so much more is possible when the various schools of Reiki work together for the benefit of the whole. We fervently hope that the Reiki techniques published here will help create more and more healing, happiness, peace and prosperity.

May your reading of this book be both entertaining and informative.

Sincerely,
Walter Lübeck and Frank Arjava Petter

What is a Technique?

—Frank Arjava Petter—

Since the lion's share of this book is dedicated to Western Reiki techniques, I would like to address the nature of these techniques in general.

Reiki itself is not a technique. After initiation into the 1st Degree energy flows completely on its own without any intervention on our part. When I am asked if we have to 'turn on' the Reiki power before using it, like a radio, I like to respond with a question of my own:

"Have you ever tried turning off the Reiki power?"

The answer is clear: Reiki is always flowing, even without us seeking to influence it. But it does flow better when we apply our intention. The techniques for the 1st, 2nd, and 3rd Reiki Degrees help us in this process. The more intensely we are involved, and this naturally applies to everything in life, the better the results will be.

The *Webster's New Universal Unabridged Dictionary* gives the origin of the word *'technique'* in this way:

—From the Greek: *technikos* = artful, skilful, specialized, expert.

—The manner and ability with which an artist, writer, dancer, athlete or the like employs the technical skills of a particular art or field of endeavor.

—The ability to apply procedures or methods so as to effect a desired result.

What Can Be Achieved with a Technique—and What Can't

In my seminars I have noticed that people are often unsure about how, where and when Reiki functions. Unfortunately some Reiki courses tend to be little more than a 'multi-level marketing business'. Graduates of these have little idea of the wonderful tools now available to them.

Regrettably many people who practice Reiki function like someone who has bought a video-recorder with no corresponding instruction booklet. They can play one cassette on it but nothing more. Groping in the dark they are left to find their own way …. Fortunately very little can go wrong in experimenting with Reiki. What can happen though is that some things do not go as we would have hoped.

So I do encourage you to experiment. Only in this way will Reiki continue to develop. If it works for you, it works! Buddha is reported to have said to his disciples:

"Truth is what works."

The incredible speed with which information is disseminated today has allowed many Reiki teachers to present material that they themselves have not yet fully understood. This is an unfortunate side of the great Reiki explosion.

The Japanese Reiki techniques that I myself uncovered in Japan have fared similarly. We began to teach these techniques only after we ourselves had practiced them for over a year and a half. It is really only possible to pass on to others what we know well. This work is being taught in many different countries now by incompetent teachers whose primary interest can only be to make money. Without the corresponding spirit such techniques are not worth a dime! They must be imbibed, lived and pulsate within the person who is teaching them. This is the only way that the spark can jump from teacher to student.

Taking Our Own Path

To explain the part that techniques play at all within the Reiki path I must back up a bit.

Techniques are a double-edged sword. They are needed in order to work effectively but the moment they begin to hinder us we must let them go. When you have crossed the river you leave the boat on the bank and continue on your way. It would be silly to carry the boat along! From this moment you follow your own path.

This applies to Reiki precisely. Find your own way and then walk it with love and humility. As you do this you need to learn to trust yourself rather than rely on others for advice. In practical terms with Reiki this means not believing anything without experimenting and trying it out for yourself. Only when you have discovered that something is true and correct on the basis of your own experience will it have value for you. No matter that well-known figures in the Reiki world may claim the opposite to be true.

The Process of Becoming a Human Being

The enlightened ones have shown us that while on the one hand we may bring certain karmic baggage into the world with us, on the other we begin our journey here on Earth pretty much as a blank page. We are not really born as human beings but only as potential human beings. We must grow into the state of being human.

Growth, they tell us, almost always occurs in connection with suffering. Especially on the spiritual path nothing is simply given to us.

The suffering that precedes awakening of consciousness is beyond moral value judgments. It is neither good nor bad. The 'good' person is rewarded by existence just as little as the 'bad' one is punished. If it were otherwise all of the prosperous and healthy people would be saints and all of the poor and sick would be sinners!

Further more existence is utterly good and compassionate. Its only concern is for our spiritual growth whatever it takes.

Karmically, however, things appear to be quite different. We reap exactly what we have sown, though the seeds may sprout in a later lifetime.

Yet the process of becoming a human being is far from fraught. Life is a game. In India they call it by the Sanskrit name *Lila*. In my experience this game seems to have three stages.

Three Phases on the Spiritual Path

The First Phase

The first phase is that of an individual who has not yet developed his ego. A person who does not know who he or she is, whose consciousness has no crystallized center cannot achieve anything much. Such an individual has no free will. He is a leaf trembling in the wind, a dream in the secrecy of his soul. He has to awaken from this dream.

This awakening is served very well by Reiki. Through the initiation into the 1st Reiki Degree we are very gently roused from our sleepy existence and given many possibilities of literally taking our life into our own hands. However we have to take this step on our own. No one, not even the most capable teacher, can propel us into taking this step.

As a 'new-born' a human being we have now taken the first step with the help of our physical body. By using the Reiki self-treatment we can now move increasingly close to our physical nature. We learn to understand our own body, learn to lovingly touch it and in the psychological sense assume more responsibility for our health and our well being. We cannot make progress without accepting responsibility for our own life.

The Second Phase

In the second phase we begin to write the book of our own life. The 2nd Reiki Degree with its techniques of distant healing treatment helps us to work on our past and future via the karma-cleansing and the affirmation.

However there is a danger in this. We can fall prey to the illusion, which would have us believe that we hold life completely in our own hands. At this point it is easy to overestimate oneself and forget one's actual state of consciousness.

During such periods of megalomania I have found a simple helpful exercise. Go out for a walk in a natural setting on a clear night and sit or lie down in a comfortable position. Up in the sky watch the stars in the firmament. Look down at yourself. Looking back up into the infinite expanse become aware of just how tiny you are, how insignificant you are. No need to judge. But recognize that you are part of the whole. Feel grateful to existence that it has given you life. Thank the universe for all the joys as well as all the difficulties that have been offered to you on your path.

The Third Phase

During the third phase we become one with everything. We now know that our individual identity is an illusion.

In order to arrive at this station however, we must first have boarded the train and left the previous stops behind us.

Once we have understood who and what we are, the behavior patterns, opinions and our own grandeur dissolve into the ocean of cosmic consciousness. Then we no longer need any type of technique or even Reiki itself.

The Reiki Initiation

—Frank Arjava Petter—

One of my favorite Zen koans is: Where does the fullness of the moon disappear to when it becomes a crescent? We all know that when the moon becomes a crescent its roundness is only temporarily concealed from our sight. It is an image that can be applied to the Reiki initiation. We human beings can only perceive what already exists, at least as a seed, in our body-mind-soul system. A computer, and our brain is a biocomputer, can only read a program that it already contains.

A Reiki initiation can be called an appeal to our Buddha nature. The mysterious thing that happens in this process has therefore always been dormant within us and waits longingly to be reawakened by a Reiki Princess or a Reiki Prince through initiation. The sole result of the initiation is that this knowledge is activated.

We can compare a Reiki initiation with the following image: Imagine that you are walking through an unfamiliar supermarket with a blindfold on your eyes. You are looking for tomatoes. You bump against the shelves, run into the walls and pick up all kinds of goods. You feel them and smell them. If you are lucky you will find the vegetable section and then it is only a matter of time before you locate the tomatoes. Once you find them the long search is over. You can go home and start cooking.

With the Reiki initiation you save yourself the searching and the bruises. During and beyond the initiation the blindfold is gently removed and you can make use of the energy whenever you like.

Adepts on the spiritual path know that just by remembering past spiritual experiences it becomes possible to re-enter those very vibrations. However this usually only functions spontaneously. If it is indulged and evoked too often it becomes a habit. The rational mind starts to ride into no-man's land on a lonely track without a driver. This way we deceive ourselves.

It is like the rats in the experiment, who repeatedly give themselves sexual orgasm to the point of utter exhaustion by triggering a contact connected to their brains. The same thing can happen to those who become addicted to spiritual experiences and initiations. So be careful!

The fertile ground of a spiritual experience is always one and the same but the experiences themselves can be very different. The person who experiences it never changes. If you focus your attention on the never changing self the arrow becomes the target!

It is after the Reiki initiation that the actual work begins. This work can only by done by each individual himself. No (Reiki) Master in the world can walk our path for us, climb our peaks or descend into our valleys. And this is also the beautiful thing about our existence. It is unique!

This book does not attempt to convey any initiation ritual or techniques. A Reiki initiation is not the same thing as a technique. Moreover, technique or ritual is only the garment and what is concealed beneath is consciousness in its purest form, or, put in another way, formlessness. What or who is concealed behind the garment is you in your essence! We all know that it can be fun to dress differently every day, but it does not change the central fact. Whatever may happen, wherever we go what we are concealing behind the garment remains the same always. It is our self.

So instead of running from one Reiki Master to the next and having ourselves initiated into this and that type of Reiki, it is

better to knuckle down to the essence. The best p?
to the essence is meditation. Dr. Mikao Usui ta?
the Reiki Gassho Meditation.

Meditating does not necessarily mean sitting like a Buoc
the lotus position under a tree until the apple falls. Everything
that we do can either be done consciously or unconsciously. Initially being meditative means doing whatever we do with as much
consciousness as we can bring to it. So the most important thing
is *how* we do something and not *what* we do.

There is a lot of good literature on the topic of meditation
especially in the cultures of Zen and Tibetan Buddhism. There
are also many capable teachers. A teacher is absolutely necessary
on this path because he or she can help us when the initial results arise. These results usually do not correspond with what
we imagined them to be or what we expected.

The next important aspect of an initiation is who is giving it
and this person's spiritual state. This has a big influence on the
outcome. An initiation given by a Lama who is authorized to
give initiations cannot be compared with an initiation received
from someone who has only read about it in a book.

Such an authorization is critical. And true initiation can only
be carried out by an individual who is fully attuned to the frequency of the energy to be transmitted. The guide needs to have
become one with it.

In all of the spiritual schools in the world a future teacher is
trained for years to acquire this ability until he or she is ready.
Even then the teacher and student may fast and meditate for
weeks before an initiation. This too will be supervised by someone who is especially experienced.

In Reiki preparation occurs somewhat more quickly because
the teacher-in-the-making has usually already been working with
the energy for a long time. Unfortunately in more recent years
the technique of the initiation has become more significant than

19

.he preparation behind it. All of us can however work precisely on this point. The ritual of the initiation is certainly important. It is a tested and well-functioning system. Just as we need our human body in order to find our self within an initiation also requires its form. In the *Heart Sutra* Buddha says: "Form is emptiness and emptiness is form." We need the form so that formlessness can manifest within it.

How to Intensify an Initiation

The basic rule for everything that we do is: Do it with your whole heart! Cook, and only cook, when you cook. Walk, and walk totally, when you go for a walk. Meditate when you meditate. We all know how difficult this really can be but it shouldn't stop us from doing the work.

We can practice being present by letting ourselves be distracted as little as possible by our inner dialogue. A simple way to practice this is to walk on a lawn very slowly, barefoot if possible.

Feel how you raise your leg in slow motion, how you take a step forward and how your foot now slowly rolls onto the grass. Step carefully onto the heel and let your foot unroll as easily and as consciously as you can. Now repeat the entire process with the other foot. Walk as slowly as possible. Every time a thought arises consciously turn to it, see it and then let it go. Don't be annoyed at these thoughts because that only makes them stronger.

We usually follow our stream of thoughts quite unconsciously and are carried off into a dream world as a result. On this dream journey we lose connection with our actual reality. In this case the reality of walking barefoot on the lawn!

An additional exercise which I personally find to be very enjoyable consists of being totally present for the person you are

speaking with in a conversation. Turn toward the person, look him or her in the eyes and banish all of your unrelated thoughts. Stay on the topic and listen to the other without judging what he or she says. See if you can be 'all ears'.

The more you can practice this way of being in the present the easier it will become to be completely present during an initiation, regardless of whether you are the 'receiver' or the 'giver'. I have put quotation marks around both words because the receiving and giving during an initiation can sometimes be suspended.

Before a Reiki Initiation

- With love prepare the room in which the initiation will take place. It should be naturally lit and freshly aired. Not everyone likes incense.

- It is also possible to do initiations outdoors. However experience has shown that it is easier for a new Reiki teacher to maintain the energy level in a closed room.

- Not everyone likes ceremonial music during the initiation either.

- If possible don't drink any alcohol the evening before. Avoid eating an excessive amount of garlic since some people find it unpleasant.

- If you smoke freshen your breath before the initiation.

- Start the initiation with an invocation. Many Reiki teachers invoke either Dr. Mikao Usui, Dr. Chujiro Hayashi, an enlightened master or a deity. This increases our consciousness of the fact that we are only a channel for the energy that is being transmitted.

- Give thanks, bowing either in front of or behind your student. Be grateful that you are being allowing to give or receive this initiation and that the other is allowing you to share this experience.

- Take every step, do every physical and mental movement with consciousness.

- Take every breath as if it were your last.

- Do not follow your thoughts into their dream world no matter how great the temptation!

What is Rainbow Reiki?

—Walter Lübeck—

Rainbow Reiki was created in the late 1980s and early '90s. The foundation on which it started to develop at that time was traditional Reiki of the Western variety as transmitted by Hawayo Takata. Traditional Japanese methods were integrated into it. Research into the roots of the 'Usui System of Natural Healing with Reiki' provided the approaches of Dr. Mikao Usui and Dr. Chujiro Hayashi. This includes the underlying spiritual wisdom such as the mystic healing practices of the Buddha Dainichi Nyorai.

Together with the traditional initiation rituals, the four symbols, their Mantras and the fundamental techniques of Reiki energy work these now form the basis of Rainbow Reiki.

Our own developments such as the essences technique, the cooperation with the Inner Child, the Higher Self and the angels, KarmaClearing and systematic chakra work came about in the course of the years. We sought continuously to facilitate healing in areas where it had not been possible to work with traditional Reiki, or at least not satisfactorily. New techniques evolved.

Rainbow Reiki naturally also takes into account a holistic approach to diet, spiritual body therapies and Feng Shui. By recognizing and normalizing imbalances in all of the important areas of life Rainbow Reiki achieves its higher degrees of effectiveness.

Just as in Mikao Usui's Reiki schools, meditation has a central place in Rainbow Reiki. With our meditation techniques it is easy to relax and regenerate. Through increasing practice of these exercises spiritual experiences and states of consciousness develop.

Anyone who learns Rainbow Reiki is simultaneously studying traditional Reiki and newly developed spiritual energy work.

These additional techniques, initiations, symbols and Mantras have been created as a result of counseling and seminar practice as well as through spiritual research.

In addition to the basic seminars for the 1st and 2nd Degree the training system of Rainbow Reiki includes a series of additional seminars such as 'Work with Power-Places and the Subtle worlds', 'Essences and Elixirs', 'Rainbow Reiki Professional Practitioner', 'Dainichi Nyorai Ki-Do' and three Master Degrees. Rainbow Reiki is taught throughout the world and hundreds of thousands of Reiki enthusiasts have been applying it for many years now.

The Reiki Healing Period

—Walter Lübeck—

Optimal Use of the Time After the Reiki Initiation

The initiation and training for a Reiki Degree can become a turning point in our lives. Extraordinary abilities can come to us in this way and are available in perpetuity and unconditionally. In addition the increase in vibrations caused by powerful initiations and energetic charging can be the lever that triggers and supports all kinds and extents of healing.

However, the way in which this 'thrust into more aliveness' manifests in each individual depends on various influencing factors. These may be largely shaped by the recipient. Yet in this process few people know what to pay attention to. Hence what follows is a summary of the most important points that I have gleaned both from my personal experience and by accompanying my Reiki students. Reiki, the spiritual life energy, has so many good things to offer. The more of us that know about it the more it may support the world during the coming global transformations .

For a start let's take a closer look at everything that can in principle be affected and moved through the Reiki initiations.

Additional Effects of the Initiations

The most important effects may well be the cleansing and the clearing as much as the triggering of healing responses on all levels.

Over the years I have perceived the individual degrees to relate to the following realms:

1ˢᵗ **Degree:** physical and emotional

2ⁿᵈ **Degree:** mental (imbalanced habits, 'stuck' ways of thinking, inflexible models of the world)

3ʳᵈ **Degree (Master/Teacher):** spiritual (clearer direction for partnership, profession and personality development. Life can become clearer and more oriented towards the themes that were laid down before birth for this specific incarnation).

These statements should not be taken as absolutes. There are often also very physical and emotional cleansing processes or corresponding healing reactions after an initiation into the 3ʳᵈ Degree. A holistically meaningful new orientation on the path of life may emerge after the 1ˢᵗ Degree and so forth. Although all of the Reiki initiations contain the same energy quality, that of Reiki, a specific focus for the individual will develop in the outcome. The personal situation of the initiate as well as the prevailing effect on specific energetic structures (for example, the chakras) and personality traits will influence this.

Moreover, a transformational shift is naturally almost always accompanied by more or less strongly accentuated clearing processes in other areas, relating directly to affected life themes.

How for example can we move to a more spiritual path in life when we are stuck in a lower vibration, disharmonious habits or blocked feelings?

The cleansings and re-orientation processes explained above may bring about the following effects:

• Chronic psychological and physical imbalances may become acute. This is similar to what can happen after intensive Reiki treatments or other holistic therapies as a healing crisis (for example: acupuncture or homeopathy).

Ethically a holistic healing calls for an enduring harmonizing of health disorders at whichever level of existence they may occur. This is not just a shifting of symptoms within the physical body to other areas of being, suppressing them or just covering up the underlying illness through some short-lived superficial balancing.

• Physical, mental and emotional stamina and capacity may diminish as a response to the initiation and even for some time afterwards. This varies according to the type and extent of the healing. Depending on the circumstances a stress level that is usually experienced as normal may be temporarily much harder to bear. Tears may even flow more easily. Feelings in general may be more readily expressed and sensitivity heightened.

Reactions to the initiations vary greatly. Some people hardly notice anything. There may still be too much resistance or such an extensive change and clearing may simply not be 'due' yet.

Cosmic influences can be very advantageous for specific areas of development. Transits, referred to by astrology as the movements of the planets through the constellations in the birth chart are a good example of this. But cosmic influences may at times also inhibit development. Some obstruction may simply be in the foreground at this time.

From the perspective of Feng Shui, environmental influences may also either encourage or retard a person's healing and development.

For this and similar reasons I have developed methods and techniques in Rainbow Reiki which are able to favorably influence the environmental conditions in a person's life allowing for complex problems to be dealt with. Important information as to how Reiki may help in allowing us to be 'moved into the light' can be found in this chapter. A topic that will also be addressed in later sections of this book.

Many people do however experience all kinds of definitive changes after Reiki initiations. Some people's entire lives change for the better within a short period of time.

People frequently report that a great many changes and much healing take place in the 21 days after an initiation. We know the story of Mikao Usui who fasted and meditated for a total of 21 days on Kurama, a holy mountain near Kyoto, to prepare for his initiation into Reiki through the creative force.

Mikao Usui, who was the founder of the Reiki System of Natural Healing, worked hard on himself through a special meditation during these three weeks. He built up such a strong resonance with Reiki within himself that he could ultimately become a permanent Reiki channel. Now however when a person is initiated into a Reiki Degree this effort is no longer necessary. The very initiation creates a lasting opening for Reiki in the initiate.

It has been my experience that there seem to be no obvious healing and growth processes in some people. Perhaps they take place deep beneath the threshold of their consciousness. Sometimes they do occur just during or shortly after the initiation. They may last a few days, weeks or in some cases even months. Nothing is wrong when there are no strong healing reactions after the initiation or when the noticeable effects only last a short time. The essential effect of the initiation is guaranteed. The enduring opening for Reiki on the three levels that are defined in the traditional degrees has been achieved.

When I refer to the Reiki healing period in this chapter I am speaking of the period of time in which an individual feels the effects mentioned above. Reiki adjusts itself to us. Life is not standardized and this applies to the effects of spiritual life energy.

Allowing the Energy of Initiations to Have Its Optimal Effect

One important point is ...

The Strength-Giving Diet

Depending on what we eat and drink, as well as how much we eat and drink, our body, mind and soul will have more or less difficulty opening to positive stimuli like Reiki. This also applies to letting go of and eliminating obstructions.

So here are some menu suggestions for the healing period after a Reiki initiation. These guidelines can of course also be used for longer Reiki treatments and anytime we want to actively contribute to a healthier way of life.

Recommended: Fresh fish (not out of a can!), steamed or briefly fried as the Asians do it. Fresh fruit and vegetables, especially: pineapples, mangos, papayas, apples, grapes, strawberries, watermelon. Ginger (also as tea) and garlic. White cabbage, potatoes, celery, green lettuce, red beets. Whole-grain products, especially: quinoa, amaranth, spelt and oats. Non-carbonated mineral water, green tea, pau d'arco tea, licorice tea and Cat's Claw tea. Noni juice. Raw-milk products. Miso, tofu and seitan. Fresh grain muesli (according to Bruker). Sauerkraut (unpasteurized). Yogurt, natural. Raw, organic cold-spun honey. Stevia (natural, very healthy sweetener). Wheat-grass juice.

Reduce: Milk products that are not made from raw milk. Meat, especially red meat. Coffee (the healthiest way to make coffee is to put a few spoons of ground coffee into a pot and then pour boiling water on it. The healthiest type of coffee is 'Organic Arabica Coffee'). Eggs. Black tea, chocolate, cocoa, nicotine (this should actually be on the 'Avoid' list but I assume that anyone who loves his smokes would rather do without the health program than the 60 daily 'smoke offerings'. But I may be wrong of course?).

Avoid: Pork and all products that contain pork such as sausage, cold cuts, lard. White, refined flour. Refined sugar. Artificial sweeteners. Soft drinks. Alcohol. Anything that comes in a can or is thoroughly denatured (such as instant soups, instant mashed potatoes, canned fruits and vegetables or canned meats). All sterilized milk products. Foods that contain chemicals like preservatives, artificial food coloring, stabilizers and taste-improving substances like MSG (look on the label for contents—you'll be amazed). Instant coffee and tea. Meals prepared in the microwave. Hardened (hydrogenized) fats and oils.

Useful Tips: If you haven't eaten fresh foods for a long time it is better not to overdo it in the beginning. In this case lightly steam or blanch foods. More than one type of fruit should not be eaten at the same time since this may cause digestive problems. Eat only freshly cooked meals, nothing that has been warmed up! Foods that have been heated more than once no longer contain vital nutrients and have very little vital energy. They are difficult to digest and burden the metabolism creating an overdose of waste materials. Eat only organic or biodynamically grown food if possible.

As a basic rule do not eat anything 'cooked' in a microwave. Whenever possible give everything that you eat and drink thirty seconds to one minute of Reiki, always after it has been heated or cooked. This increases its energetic value aiding and improving the digestion and metabolism.

Pray and Eat Better: With a little prayer you can do something for your spiritual development and effectively improve the energetic value of your food at the same time. Simply think or say: "I thank everyone who has contributed to this meal." During the prayer center your attention on your heart chakra and direct it into the food. The effect of this beneficial exercise in gratitude can also be checked with a pendulum or the kinesiology arm test. Test the charging of your food's vital energy before and directly after the prayer. You will experience a very pleasant surprise! You can of course apply the same test when you treat food or drink with Reiki.

Pleasant Relaxation Exercises

Allow yourself regular Reiki treatments and pay attention to the results. For example, how does your body react, how do your moods change and what kinds of daydreams arise? It's a good idea to keep a journal on this.

Meditation, guided imagery, breath exercises and autogenic training can effectively complement your Reiki sessions. In the healing period after a Reiki initiation it is very important to rest and thereby create the necessary space for the increased activity of the body's own power to heal itself.

Take time to feel yourself. Take yourself seriously! Allow yourself to express moods and let your feelings flow. Be honest with yourself and contemplate your life up to now. What are you content with? What are you not?

Which people you know strengthen you and help you to find yourself and stand up for yourself? Which people do you feel tend to have the opposite effect? Decide for yourself and put a priority on contact with those from whom you benefit. This does not mean that you have to hold the same opinion as these people. It is often a special sign of friendship to address things that others don't have the self-confidence to talk about.

Here is a simple and very effective relaxation exercise that I like to use myself:

Search your memory for three situations where you have been very relaxed and happy. Take notes on these experiences including what you have seen, heard, smelled, tasted and physically felt. Underline the sensory perceptions that especially promoted or triggered these feelings. Such impressions are also called key perceptions.

During these minutes, which should be undisturbed, imagine yourself in each experience and focus your attention especially on the key factors that really cause your heart to rejoice. They evoke deep relaxation, a sense of security, fulfillment, strength and a healthy sense of self and happiness within. While you are doing this place your hands intuitively on areas of the body so that Reiki can give additional help wherever it may be needed.

Try out the various situations a few times until you notice which of them has the greatest possible effect on you. If you discover that some of the selected memories are not optimal drop them and find more suitable ones and work with them instead.

However, do not change without a reason! Unnecessary change forces this process to start over again each time. Your subconscious mind will be more open from one time to the next for work with the imagination. Thus the effects will be varied and more or less intense.

This combined exercise can bring you relief in no time at all, especially after a strenuous day at work: About 20 minutes is all that is needed to recuperate and gather fresh strength, distancing yourself from the stresses of everyday life. At the same time you will recreate the desire to engage in dynamic leisure activities. Many people who would otherwise have just enough energy for a dreary evening of TV (after work) become 'fit for fun' again with the help of this simple technique.

In this exercise pay particular attention to the region from the navel to the solar plexus beneath the sternum, the abdomen as well as the temples. When there has been a lot of tension with other people the heart and throat chakras as well as the kidneys are often grateful for an extra dose of Reiki.

Balancing Movement

Extensive walks, light aerobic* running, gymnastics, Yoga, tai chi, the Five Tibetans™, qigong and similar non-competitive sports activities gently stimulate the lymphatic system and the flow of the forces in the subtle energy body. Thus they support the comprehensive detoxification, purification and regeneration processes stimulated by the initiations and the Reiki treatments. Reiki cannot replace movement since the body consists largely of material components. They need exercise in order not to 'rust'. It is important to increase the demands placed on the body slowly. In no case should it have excessive demands placed upon it.

Health-Promoting Lifestyle during the Reiki Healing Period

Plenty of sleep, at least eight hours every night. The sleep before midnight is especially important. Go to bed by 10 p.m. at the latest! Reduce stress as much as possible. Talk with friends when you have something to share. Perhaps consult an oracle to get in tune with new directions, new openings.

---

* 'Aerobic' implies that you do not get out of breath. Your body is filling up with oxygen as long as you move so that your breath deepens pleasantly. As long as you don't have to gasp to recover from a run the tissues are fairly flooded with this elixir of life. The metabolism improves. It helps lose weight and strengthens the immune system. In addition oxygenation prevents chronic diseases like cancer.
Reiki optimally integrates this positive 'input' into the metabolism if you give yourself a treatment after working out. Professor von Ardenne and Professor van Aaken have done important research on the health-promoting effects of oxygen. Many good publications by each of them are available.

Some Examples of Important Questions for the Oracle:

1. What should I change in my life so that I can be more in tune with the cosmic order and my life's plan?
2. What can I do to open up more in my (a) partnership with regard to the cosmic order and my life's plan?
3. What can I do so that my professional work is more and more in keeping with the cosmic order and my life's plan?
4. What can I do to improve (stabilize) my health in a holistic sense?
5. What should I change in myself so as to live and work more harmoniously and constructively with my family (or: my friends, my colleagues)?
6. What is my greatest block in relation to the holistically meaningful use of my Reiki abilities?
7. How can I resolve this block?
8. What can I do to love my inner child more, better understanding and respect its needs?
9. How can I make my body happier?

Over the years working on these questions tarot cards, runes, *Chakra Energy Cards,* or the *I Ching* have proved very helpful in my counseling practice.

It is, of course, also possible to meditate on all of these questions.

Clarifying Attention

What kinds of dreams do you have? Keep a dream journal if you wish to delve more deeply into this topic.

What do you continuously encounter in your everyday life that relates to the healing period after a Reiki initiation?

What thoughts recur frequently?

Which animals, plants and stones do you come across time and again or in specific situations that are meaningful for you?

Read about helper forces that have been sent to you so that you can more easily learn to understand their messages.

Meditate on these themes and also ask an oracle.

Being in Harmony with the People around You

Ask your family and your friends to be understanding about what is happening for you during your Reiki healing period. Explain to them that there are many changes going on in you at the moment and that you may require more time than usual for yourself. Let them know that you may be more sensitive and vulnerable than they normally know you to be.

In no case should you attempt to 'preach' to your fellow human beings. If someone wants to try out Reiki, well and good. Otherwise it's best to look after your own affairs. Your friends and relatives don't necessarily have to share your interests and it's really enough if they respect your activities and viewpoints, and you respect theirs. Tolerance and the exchange of personal points of view and preferences in a respectful constructive manner are a good foundation for genuine deep love to grow upon.

If folks get on your nerves with their 'materialism' and their 'callousness' retreat a bit and make it clear to yourself that they are not the cause of your increased sensitivity. It will not remain this extreme for very long.

In these situations you can see how committed you are to your spiritual path. Instead of demanding that the other person change, use your knowledge and abilities to grow out of your own problems. This path may be long and essentially strenuous but changes that occur in this way are truly for the better.

Sometimes separations may be the result of the consciousness-expanding processes triggered by Reiki. When the paths of two people no longer fit together it is important to respect lovingly this also. However, if at all possible you should not make major decisions when a storm of emotions is raging. It is better to wait until the waves have subsided and you feel centered again. In a harmonious mood you can think things through thoroughly. This way you can make those decisions that will bring you closer to the light.

Reiki Treatments

You can certainly also give others Reiki during your healing period. Reiki flows to everything that you touch. Yet stay consciously with yourself all through this important time of transformation, it is primarily about you. You are now very important. There are people who have passed up the opportunity for their own healing and re-orientation by being too concerned about the care of others. Remember, those seeking help can also go to others for advice and assistance. If you now use the opportunity to take advantage of the process you will also have more to offer later.

Give yourself a whole-body treatment at least three times a week for one to two months after your initiation into a Reiki Degree. Aren't you worth it?! And if you say "no" then why not? The healing period after an initiation is blessed. Through the Reiki Degree you have received a wonderful set of tools. Are you going to stack them in the corner with the other things you once 'achieved' and then quickly forgot, even though they really could have changed your life for the better ? What would you say to a good friend who goes on acquiring wonderful things but lets them gather dust unused? If this applies to you ask an oracle about it. (also see page 288, *"The Chakra Energy Cards"*).

Many people who have been initiated into Reiki do not actualize their own potential. They either fail to use this fantastic force or only make it available to others. This is a great waste but it is never too late to learn. Reiki can do wonders for you right now. Just simply say "yes" to the light and to love!

Perhaps you would like to use this as a small but potant exercise.

It goes like this: Stand in front of a mirror. Look yourself in the face and smile. Now say, "From the bottom of my heart I say 'yes' to the light and to love. From the bottom of my heart I say 'yes' to myself and to my spiritual path. I am special. The creative force loves me just as I am. It has let me become as I am and wants to make something very special possible that is good for me and for the entire world."

Now smile at yourself and bow before you go.

Do this brief exercise every evening for a month before going to bed. It has already helped many people change their self-image and thereby give their life a new and positive direction.

Art can be so healing. Discover the artist inside you! Paint a picture during the week before the initiation. Do this very spontaneously letting it come out however you feel. Paint another picture during the week after the seminar and a third at the end of your healing period. Look at all three pictures only after a month has passed. Meditate on each of them.

Guest Initiations: What Happens when a Person Is Initiated More Than Once into a Reiki Degree?

Since the Reiki abilities of a given degree have already been awakened and stabilized for you, additional initiations essentially have the effect of a strengthener sometimes even of a trigger for overdue processes of cleansing and re-orientation. Because most people who practice Reiki regularly see their perceptivity for subtle vibrations increase over time, 'guest initiations' are often more intense than the first initiation.

Sometimes the additional (usually short-term) sensitization caused by a second initiation is seen as an intensification of Reiki abilities. This is not necessarily the case. A temporarily intensified indirect activation of the heart and forehead chakras may result however. This can allow more easy opening up to clients on the emotional level. Compassion, warm-heartedness and emotional warmth become intensified.

Since Reiki is better absorbed by the body of a recipient when this person feels more completely accepted, more will now happen than before. Whether or not this state endures depends upon the willingness of the person to continue working on the improvement of these qualities in their everyday life and in the underlying mental and emotional conditioning.

During the healing period after guest initiations there are rarely such extensive and far-reaching reactions as after the first initiation into that degree.

Pitfalls along the Way

At this point I feel it is important to mention some of the convictions that can impede the use of the transforming, loving power of Reiki initiations and treatments. It is not so difficult to recognize these obstacles and avoid them.

Pitfall No. 1: The initiation and or Reiki treatment solves my problems, allows my personality to mature and automatically supports my spiritual development without any other effort on my part.

This approach blocks development of personal happiness. It is practically a guarantee that Reiki initiations and treatments will not have their essential effect. On the contrary Reiki promotes life processes, it is the fundamental effect of this force. But if we do not want to become more alive in some way in order to avoid the need to assume more responsibility or make unpalatable decisions, we may unconsciously adopt such a path and do nothing more.

Furthermore, frequent contact with the spiritual life energy while simultaneously refusing to follow the direction it provides can lead us into unpleasant, tense situations.

On the one hand Reiki will not force us to be happy. Our body draws Reiki because deep down we want to be whole and happy. On the other hand some conscious or unconscious forces resist and would prefer to remain in the familiar prison of conventional viewpoints and life structures. The concrete consequences of such contradictions may manifest as sleep problems, nervousness, irritability and general feelings of ill health.

Reiki, whether given in the form of an initiation or a treatment promotes our material efforts to find happiness and become healthy and successful. When we do not make this effort there is nothing that can come of it. If this success is sought in a way that is not at all appropriate for us, Reiki cannot do much more than draw our attention to the dead-end we have landed ourselves in. This is why a thorough rethink, new decisions and new actions are necessary to live life in a way that truly corresponds with our own real needs.

Pitfall No. 2: I must have as many initiations as possible and reach the next higher Reiki Degree as soon as possible because everything in my life will be easier then.

This does not correspond with what really happens. No matter what degree we have ourselves initiated into, the important thing is always what we do with our new possibilities.

The initiation itself presents many possibilities. What these are and how to use them constructively is learned in the corresponding training. This should always be in a personal encounter which usually occurs in the form of a seminar. Although books can provide many impulses, useful knowledge and insights they cannot and should not replace the direct person-to-person relationship with the Reiki teacher.

This has many advantages from the spiritual perspective. Personal development evolves in this way since love and forgiveness, tolerance and respect, gratitude and sincerity, friction and reconciliation cannot be learned via theory. After all, this and other profoundly human qualities are the field of activity for Reiki, the healing spiritual life energy. It does help us be happy, whole and successful in our everyday life and in relating with the people who are involved with us.

The initiation and the training into the art of Reiki give us the tools that we need. The individual initiations and training stages of the Reiki system offer each of us wonderful possibilities and fascinating experiences. Together they create what Reiki is. An old proverb says that all good things come in threes. We should not underestimate the potential of each individual degree.

This book offers you a little insight into the many possibilities that Reiki brings. However the emphasis here is upon *little*. It would be no problem to put together a one-year seminar on the 1ˢᵗ Degree that contains no repetitions. The same applies to both of the further degrees as well. New things can be continuously learned from Reiki with much gain throughout an entire lifetime.

We, your two authors, have both practiced Reiki for more than a decade and are constantly learning how it can be applied in new and even better, more comprehensive, flexible, spiritual and powerful ways. Life is learning and it is wonderful!

Pitfall No. 3: The more I am involved with Reiki the happier I will become.

This also misses the point. Like everything else our occupation with Reiki should be in a healthy balanced relationship with other activities. It is certainly normal for us to be full of enthusiasm for a few weeks after a Reiki seminar with our thoughts focused mainly on this wonderful gift. But at some point other aspects of our life will take up their importance once again. Only like this our Reiki practice can help harmonize all the areas of our life and support our development.

Reiki is not life, Reiki promotes life. Whatever Reiki touches inside will be healed when we integrate it into our life. Balance and flow are the foundations of happiness. In the East this has been expressed for thousands of years in the laws of yin and yang.

I hope that these insights into the 'secrets of the Reiki healing period' will help you on your path. I suggest that you refer back to this chapter often. Take notes, think about the statements and try out the suggestions. With this approach there is much for you to gain. Even if some aspects of what I am sharing here seem superfluous or exotic at the moment, these impulses have developed from a Reiki practice that began in 1987. They have brought much good to a great many people. They will also support you on your way if you give them a chance.

Is Reiki an Intelligent Force that Can Do no Wrong?

—Walter Lübeck—

A great many enthusiasts of Reiki wonder about this. It is important to understand precisely what Reiki can do on its own and what the Reiki practitioner must pay attention to. This is the only way that the spiritual life energy can develop its full effect.

This statement that Reiki is always absorbed by the recipient is fundamentally true. The following guidelines should be taken into consideration individually:

• The body consciousness of the client (Inner Child) must trust the practitioner and feel safe and accepted in the treatment situation. Loving behavior, understanding and empathy, sincerity and gentleness can open many doors, not just for Reiki.

• This body consciousness must be willing to give up its imbalances. If it places value on maintaining an illness Reiki will not have a noticeable effect in the beginning. In such a case supplemental measures have to be used to get the subconscious mind to comprehend the necessity for change and to motivate it to heal. Some people unconsciously use their health problems as a substitute for constructive meaning in their life or to gain attention and special treatment. As understandable as this may be, especially when someone's life story has been characterized by great suffering, it is absolutely necessary for them to let go of the illness and learn to obtain the benefit it seems to provide in other more constructive ways. In this step as well this range of Reiki techniques can be of great help.

• Reiki always promotes living processes. Among these are detoxification and purification on all levels of body, mind and soul.

Assistance must be provided especially when healing such extensive imbalances.

For example this could be expressed in a healthy diet, aerobic movement, counseling or stress releasing forms of expression such as painting, dancing, singing, sculpting, writing and even massages. It is imperative to drink enough fresh, non-carbonated water. Depending on the climate and the extent of physical activity the following rule of thumb applies: 30 to 40 ml of water per kilogram of body weight daily.

If the healing reactions are too intense or unpleasant congestion occurs from dissolving blocks like headache or nausea, these can be resolved or avoided entirely through the correct application of Reiki. Appropriate grounding measures as well as chakra and brain hemisphere balancing are especially useful for the latter.

• Reiki sessions can be optimally tailored to the individual needs of every client through knowledge of material and subtle anatomy, the physiology of the human body as well as via psychosomatic and spiritual correlations.

• Depending on how Reiki is used a greater or lesser degree of healing becomes possible. This depends on whether or not it is given systematically on the meridians, major and secondary chakras, reflex zones, organs and mental-emotional areas in a way that is connected to the client's personal problems. Without some sort of framework it will be less effective.

Physical complaints frequently require karmic harmonization or a change in the way a person thinks and lives in order for either a cure or alleviation to occur.

While Reiki always works in the direction that life is going, this does not diminish the Reiki practitioner's responsibility for its proper application.

Since the very beginning the emphasis in Reiki has been on the responsibility of the practitioner to offer the broadest possible range of healing. Dr. Mikao Usui and Dr. Chujiro Hayashi trained their students in a great variety of ways to treat people, teaching them to perceive energetic imbalances so that they could provide focused and effective treatment with the spiritual life energy. In his courses Dr. Chujiro Hayashi distributed written material on the causes of common diseases so that his students could more easily find the appropriate treatment sequences. More extensive information and explanations of the traditional Reiki treatment techniques of Dr. Mikao Usui and Dr. Chujiro Hayashi can be found in our book *The Spirit of Reiki* (by Lübeck/Petter/Rand, Lotus Press/Shangri-La).

Anyone who uses Reiki, or any other type of healing method for that matter, and sloughs off the responsibility for the results onto God, his higher self, some guardian angel or anyone else is acting with negligence. Reiki is a wonderful force. We should honor it by using it as effectively as possible for the benefit of everyone and assume the responsibility.

I think it's obvious that a prayer for spiritual assistance during a healing needs to accompany our limited human efforts. A spiritual healer always acts in keeping with the principle: "I constantly do the best that I can and fervently ask the creative force to complete my imperfect efforts through its blessing and its wisdom."

People frequently ask how they can use Reiki to protect themselves from one thing or another. How can we protect ourselves against the 'negative' energy of other people? How can we strengthen our aura, protect our house or prevent anything 'negative' from happening?

My first response to these questions is that there is nothing that is 'negative'. There are things and people in our surroundings that feel unpleasant to us. There may be any number reasons for this and it's best to not even try to analyze it but simply to say that someone or something is not compatible with you. They simply do not vibrate at the same frequency as you do.

The very idea that we must protect ourselves is to take a step in the wrong direction. Whatever we fear has power over us. Fear indicates that we are separated from our surroundings. This is perhaps the greatest folly that we human beings can commit with our minds.

Fear paralyses our creativity, our joy in life and our potential to live life to its fullest. The tragedy is that fear opens us to all the various impacts of negativity. If we are afraid of a psychic attack this opens our receptivity to it. If we are afraid of an accident we may drive with such distraction that we actually do become involved in an accident.

However fear in a dangerous situation can also save one's life. Fear as a natural state is a blessing and the art is to look it in the face. Then the tiger often turns back into a stuffed animal on its own!

But unbased feelings of fear are like a neon light. They attract what is feared with much noise and fuss. An affirmation such as: "I am safe and protected" chains our consciousness to the fear of being unsafe and unprotected. Without the clearing and harmonization of fears and their individually related problems, protection measures like wearing amulets, reciting Mantras or hanging up pictures of saints only create the opposite effect.

How to Get Off the Train of Fear

The simplest method is to just say "no" and let this decision help you to get off at the first stop. When I feel that someone is psychically attacking me I say within myself:

"This does not belong to me, this is not my responsibility." I neither protect myself with Reiki nor with any other method, nor do I send the 'negative energy' back to its sender. So I do not defend myself against it. I simply let it flow through me and that's it! To do this I must have absolute trust in myself. I must be self-confident and have a good deal of self-love. This topic will be addressed again later, under "Techniques."

However, until you have either learned to transform negative energy or to allow it to flow through you, the Reiki techniques in this book that are concerned with protection measures are a good aid. Use them to strengthen your aura and your immune system. Learn to stand on your own two feet and then remember that they are only crutches that you can later discard.

Before, during, and After a Reiki Treatment

—Frank Arjava Petter—

Instructions for the Reiki Practitioner:

- Wash your hands with clean cold water.
- Rinse your mouth out with clean water. If you smoke or have eaten something with a strong smell use a mouthwash or mints, etc.
- Drink a glass of clean water.
- Take off all of your metal jewelry: watches (especially quartz watches), rings, belts, etc. Metal, especially when it closes around a part of the body like a ring or a bracelet can negatively affect the natural flow of energy.
- Ask your client to do likewise.
- Spend a few minutes talking with your client. Ask their reason for coming to you, whether there is pain or other complaints and the date of the last thorough medical examination.
- In case you are not familiar with your client's illness look it up in a pathology handbook. Be sure you have one on hand.
- Ask the client about family background, work, etc. Without pressuring the client you can often get quite an exact picture of the situation.
- Briefly explain to the client what to expect during the treatment.
- Explain that during the treatment it is possible that feelings previously banished to the depths will come to light and that it is okay to experience these feelings and to express them.

- If possible allow your client a few minutes after the treatment to regain composure.
- Do not send him home right away, and especially not directly onto the freeway! At least 15 minutes of rest is always appropriate.
- Change the sheets after the treatment.
- Wash your hands again with clean cold water.
- Allow yourself a few minutes of rest before you receive your next client.

Instructions for the Reiki Client:

- If possible come to the treatment rested and freshly showered. The more awake you are the better you will be able to respond to and enjoy the treatment.
- Tell the person giving the treatment why you have come. If you have problems talk about them.
- Be as relaxed as possible. Breathe deeply and calmly.
- Trust the person giving you the treatment.
- Dedicate the time of the treatment to your body and your health with complete consciousness.
- Do not 'help' the Reiki practitioner during the treatment. If for example, he wants to place a hand under your back let him do it alone. You should now be totally relaxed.
- If you feel pain or a (perhaps unfamiliar) strong flow of energy mention this to the practitioner.
- When feelings come up from the deep inside let this happen even if they are unpleasant. If you need to cry or laugh let this happen. If it is very unpleasant for you try to alert the practitioner.

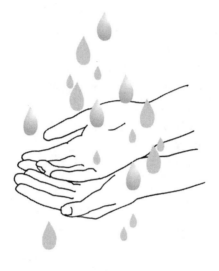

Wash your hands with clean cold water

How I Use the Reiki-Symbols

—Frank Arjava Petter—

In this chapter I would like to explain briefly how I use the Reiki symbols of the 2nd and 3rd Degrees. There are basically no right or wrong ways to apply them. The most important thing is to find a way of working that suits you personally.

We learn most effectively with the help of our senses. These I divided into three main groups. It's obvious that every human being uses each of these senses but the individual will normally have one sense more strongly developed than the others. Each of us belongs primarily to one of these groups:

1. Feeling, kinesthetic (this group includes the sense of touch as well as those of taste and smell)

2. Auditory

3. Visual

To discover which group you belong to close your eyes briefly and ask yourself which sense you use most extensively to perceive the world around you. For example, do you listen to your partner's voice to know how he or she is doing or can you see this by simply looking? Or do you perhaps even feel it as you walk in the door?

You can make good use of this knowledge when you work with the Reiki symbols. First check the list below for the various ways to work with the symbols to find out which one appears to be the easiest for you. Working with the Reiki symbols of course mainly focuses on mastering the written symbols. Naturally this would be hard to do with one's sense of hearing!

Once you have mastered working with the symbols you can begin to activate your other senses more fully. If you are like me and not very visually inclined you can use visualization exercises to help you expand your horizon. If your sense of touch is not very strong take into your hands various objects that you like and feel them. If your hearing is not particularly acute imagine sounds that you like to hear and practice this.

Here is the list with the techniques:
- Write the symbol with one hand and mentally repeat it three times (Feeling, kinesthetic).
- Write the symbol with your inner eye and repeat it mentally three times (visual).
- Write the symbol with your head or your entire body and repeat it three times in your mind (Feeling, kinesthetic).
- Project the symbol with your inner eye like a slide and mentally repeat it three times (visual).
- Write the symbol with the tip of your tongue on the roof of your mouth and mentally repeat it three times (Feeling, kinesthetic).
- Write the symbol with your hand or a finger on the part of the body to be treated and mentally repeat it three times (Feeling, kinesthetic).
- Write the symbol in one of the above-described ways and let it flow out of your hands during the treatment (Feeling, kinesthetic).
- Project the symbol with your eyes onto the targeted part of the body and mentally repeat it three times (visual).
- If you are working with a client who has already been initiated into Reiki 2 you can also say the Mantra out loud (auditory).

The same rule always applies: Write the symbol once and then mentally repeat the Mantra three times.

In Japanese Reiki system of Dr. Mikao Usui and Dr. Chujiro Hayashi the Mantras of the power symbol and the mental-healing symbol are not spoken out loud. They are simply regarded as the names of the symbols.

When we met with Ms. Yamaguchi in Kyoto in the summer of 2000 she said as we spoke about the symbols: "Repeating the Mantras is like taking a spoon in your hand and saying 'spoon, spoon, spoon'!"

We all laughed heartily. But this caused me to think deeply about the Mantras afterwards.

The work with the Reiki symbols has been very strongly emphasized in the Western tradition. Through constant repetition the Mantras have developed a life of their own which we should put to use.

Everyone has certain habits. These habits are either of a physical, mental or emotional nature. When we repeat a certain action over and over it becomes habitual. The same naturally also applies to our thoughts and feelings.

The way we use the word habit seems to leave a bad aftertaste because we mostly connect it with negative activities. However this does not tell the whole story. We can also develop positive habits. My spiritual master Osho has said that any action we want to turn into a habit demands only 60 minutes of practice. If you drink tea for at least 60 minutes every day as I do, you will become a 'tea-junkie' within a few weeks. If you meditate every day for an hour this will also become a habit. This is *not* a bad habit!

The use of the Reiki symbols and the corresponding Mantras can become habitual if we use them every day. The more you work with the symbols the more successful you become. The old proverb says: 'Practice makes perfect'. Just as you have to train a muscle to get it into optimal shape so it can help you in your work, you also have to train to work with the symbols. The possibilities are infinite. So let's get started!

Every time you say one of the Mantras in your mind or out loud it gains in power. It is important always to say the Mantras with resolution and force. As soon as they are solidly anchored in your mind, and experience has shown that this usually occurs within several months, it will be enough simply to repeat the Mantra to manifest the specific energy.

An anecdote from my own life illustrates this. A few years ago I drove a rental car along a typical English country road. It was bordered by hedges that were maybe three feet high. Suddenly a suicidal pheasant shot out of the hedge directly in front of my car. Since I have been a vegetarian for twenty years or more I wasn't interested in roasting it for dinner. It was too late to think, let alone apply the brakes. Before I knew it I had roared out the Mantra of the power symbol. It came out very loud and powerfully like a command from an Emperor. And as if it had been propelled by a rocket the pheasant flew back into the hedge.

Even today I am still grateful to the Emperor for his help and I am certain that the pheasant feels the same way!

Note: It is possible that at some point you may catch yourself performing a distant healing treatment without the help of the Reiki symbols. The symbols primarily help us in focusing our mind and energy like a laser beam onto a specific point or person. Once you have internalized this it is possible that you no longer need any aids. I don't want to make any rules out of my personal experience but I use the Reiki symbols to send energy however it comes up. Sometimes symbols, sometimes not.

Feng Shui*
during the Reiki Session

—Walter Lübeck—

A positive atmosphere in the room can contribute a lot to the success of a Reiki session. This chapter contains some tips to consider.

Firstly be sure you are not giving the treatment in the direct vicinity of a fuse box, electrical devices, wall sockets or close to a power line. Likewise avoid working near a wall that has any electrical fields in it or on the other side. There is evidence that electric radiation disturbs the body's natural ability to regulate itself. At best it weakens the immune system and prevents relaxation.

If the vicinity of an electrical device or power line cannot be avoided a large-scale Rainbow Reiki shower should be created above the treatment space. This will stabilize your client's state as well as your own since both are then enveloped in an intensified field of spiritual life energy. A thorough cleansing of the room before the session is a good practice.

According to the teachings of Feng Shui the edges of walls or furniture that point to the place where the Reiki session is to happen radiate sha. This is an unhealthy form of *qi* (life energy) because it is very concentrated and flows too directly in straight lines. Stress, tensions, feebleness, weakening of the body's own

---

*Feng Shui is an art and a science that is thousands of years old. It involves designing living spaces and gardens in such a way that their material and energetic spacial arrangements promote health, success, happiness, vitality and a sense of well being. The inhabitants are thus protected against problematic outside effects.

immune systems, nervousness and irritability as well as head-aches and many other symptoms can be triggered by spending a long period of time where *sha* is radiating. Once the room has been deeply cleansed cover these edges with scarves or the like secured with thumbtacks or adhesive tape.

The room should be thoroughly aired before the session but be sure that it is pleasantly warm. People do cool down easily during a treatment with Reiki. Stimulated by the spiritual life energy the body's own energy system switches from the active to the passive state. The active state is needed to confront the world and to protect against disharmonious environmental influences. The passive state however allows recuperation, healing and regeneration even if the body's ability to protect itself against changing environmental conditions is weaker. Thus the temperature in the room should be pleasantly warm, without any drafts.

If you would like to use incense always ask your client first. They could be allergic to it so offer a 'sample sniff' so that the room is not filled with a fragrance your client does not like. Incense should always be used sparingly.

If other people live on the premises let them know that you don't want to be disturbed during the session. A sign on the door: 'Please Do Not Disturb—Reiki Session in Progress' should do the trick.

Natural lighting is always preferred. Please do not use neon tubes since their radiation is disharmonious. Halogen lamps are also not advisable. A healthier light is created by regular incandescent light bulbs or better yet, natural candles which are known to create a very beautiful warm atmosphere.

Music can contribute to the harmony of a Reiki session, especially when outside noises penetrate. If you do play music take your client's tastes into consideration and keep the volume where it aids the session.

Reiki sessions should not take place in a room with damp or moldy walls. If no other space is available cleanse the room intensely and create Rainbow Reiki showers to make the most of your situation.

The Techniques
(In Alphabetical Order)

The following section of this book presents a large collection of techniques that have proved valuable in practice.

Please read the explanations carefully and take time to try out the exercises. Use them to work on the practical problems of your everyday life. While you are learning to use them don't start with the most difficult ones. Check the results that you have achieved. A combination of various techniques is often very successful.

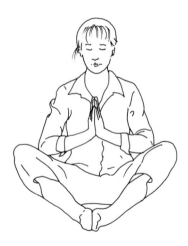

Arm-Muscle Test from Applied Kinesiology

Prerequisite:

A Reiki initiation is not necessary for the successful use of this technique. The kinesiology arm-test is used in Rainbow Reiki as a diagnostic tool* to make the energy work with Reiki more effective.

Technical Instructions

Two people, called the Tester (T) and Client (C) here, are required for this test. Although this version of the kinesiology arm-test is simplified it is still more than adequate for everyday situations. If you would like to attain more precise results consult the related literature and attend some of the kinesiology seminars now being offered in most cities.

Preparation for T and C: Drink a glass of either mineral water or filtered energetically activated tap water (non-carbonated). Remove any quartz watches, closed metal chains and metal rings. Gently tap the thymus gland in the rhythm of the heartbeat. This gland is located above the sternum between the heart and the bottom of the throat. For three minutes allow Reiki to be absorbed at the positions 1 (face) and 2 (temples) of the whole-body treatment. It is best to assume a mental attitude of 'let's see what will happen'. Bias interferes with the test! Don't ask any questions about future events, life, death or pregnancy. If there are particularly strong ten-

---

* In this context diagnosis should not be understood in the medical sense but as a method for determining a person's reactions to certain perceptions, substances, memories, people, feelings, types and amounts of energy.

sions between partners they should do the arm test with someone else with whom they have a more neutral relationship.

Calibration: T and C stand facing each other. C places the palm of the muscularly weaker arm (recipient hand) on her own thymus gland and holds the other arm horizontally out to the side at shoulder-height. T places one hand on the shoulder of the weaker arm of C and a finger of the other hand on the side of the elbow just behind the wrist of C's outstretched stronger arm. T says: "Hold!" and presses it down for about five seconds with gradually increasing pressure. While doing this he notes the resistance offered

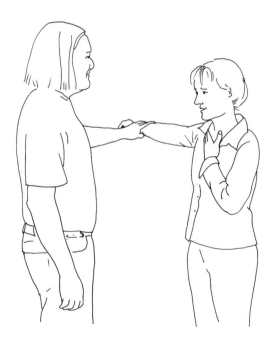

The arm test from applied kinesiology

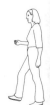

by C who is trying to keep her arm up, against the pressure, with all her might. This test shows the momentary basic strength.

Now the actual test can be done.

Test: The process is principally the same as the one described above under 'Calibration'. The only difference is the positioning of C's recipient hand. It is placed on the thymus gland for testing questions. To test the chakras, it is positioned about one handwidth from the respective energy center with the inside of the hand facing the body. To test material objects it is placed on the thymus gland or the navel and the object to be tested is held between the palm of the hand and the body.

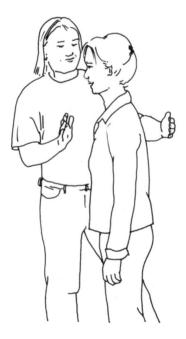

Treating a chakra with the dancing hands technique

Animals—Treating with Reiki 1

Prerequisite:

1st Reiki Degree

Technical Instructions

Step 1: If the animal is large enough place your hands on the area of the body that you would like to treat. The organs of animals are arranged similarly to those of human beings. For small animals you can cover some or even all of the inner organs with one hand position.

Step 2: The animal specifies the length of the treatment. As soon as it becomes restless you know that the end of the treatment is approaching. My cat immediately takes to its heels when it has had enough of my Reiki hands.

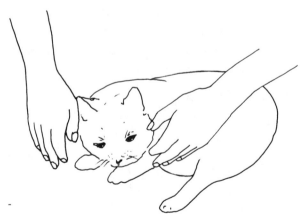

The cat determines the length of the treatment

Length	As with human beings, 20 to 60 minutes and longer if necessary. Otherwise until the animal becomes restless and leaves on its own accord.
Please Note	Reiki does not replace the vet. In cases of infectious and life-threatening illnesses, it is absolutely necessary to consult a qualified veterinarian.
Use	This technique can help in the treatment of an animal of any size, from an ant to a zebra.
Combination	Distant healing treatment, if you cannot touch the animal treat it with one of the distance-treatment techniques (see pages 121-148).
Philosophy	In the interview with Dr. Mikao Usui published in *Reiki—The Legacy of Dr. Usui* he holds that humans are the most highly developed beings in existence and that the Reiki force flows through people for the good of the whole. This suggests that everything in this universe is related to everything else in some mysterious way and an invisible bond connects each one of us with all of life. When I notice a suffering animal I send it Reiki. Thus I become involved in the life and death of this living being and in this way assume full responsibility for my actions.

What Works? What Doesn't?

The suffering of animals may be relieved in this way and they are grateful for it.

Animals like Reiki. I have had many wonderful experiences treating dogs, cats, horses, cows, birds and all kinds of small animals that were a success all round.

The most important thing in dealing with animals is to love them and not be afraid of them. We can use distance Reiki to work on any fears we may have surrounding animals by addressing related childhood traumas.

Anyone who does not like animals and has no plans of becoming an animal-lover would be safer leaving their treatment to someone else. So if you belong to this group stay out of the lion's cage!

Experiences
I had a funny experience several years ago. I was relaxing on a beach on Lake Michigan with a few friends when two large flies paid me a visit. Rather than chase them away I took a thin branch, let Reiki flow and began to train them. Within a few minutes the flies were walking up and down on the branch like super-models. A short time later they even let me pet them!

Animals—Treating with Reiki 2

Prerequisite:

2nd Reiki Degree

Technical Instructions

Step 1: Stand or sit in a relaxed manner with both feet parallel to each other and take several deep breaths.

Step 2: Draw the distance-treatment symbol once in the way that is most comfortable for you and mentally repeat the corresponding Mantra three times.

Step 3: Repeat the name for the species of the animal to be treated three times. For example, say: "eagle, eagle, eagle …."

Step 4: Send the mental-healing symbol to the animal.

Step 5: Seal everything with the power symbol (as usual draw it once and repeat the Mantra of the symbol three times).

Step 6: If you would like to add emphasis say once only: "With the help of the Reiki symbol I am now sending the healing Reiki energy to this animal. May this energy do whatever is best for its highest good."

Step 7: Now treat either the injured parts of the body of the animal or give it a whole-body treatment. You can also let your breath flow into the treatment.

Length   The same as for human beings, 20 to 60 minutes and longer if necessary. Otherwise until the animal becomes restless and leaves on its own accord.

Please Note Reiki does not replace the vet. In cases of infectious and life-threatening illnesses it is absolutely necessary to consult a qualified veterinarian doctor.

Use   This technique can be used to heal animals that either cannot be touched for reasons of safety or because they are somewhere else.

Combination Treatment of animals with the 1st Reiki Degree, treatment of feed or drinking water with the 1st or 2nd Reiki Degree, Rainbow Reiki essences.

Philosophy   Animals cannot ask for help, particularly wild animals. In this case we must decide what is best for the animal and our own health in the moment.

What Works? What Doesn't?

We can help an animal with distance Reiki as long as we observe the same preconditions as for distance Reiki with a human client. A single treatment can be very successful but most cases require treating the animal at least once a day for a week. Reiki is not a miracle drug!

Experiences Last year I was visiting friends in New Zealand when their ducklings hatched. One of the little newborns was very weak and I feared that it would not survive its first day. I took the duckling in my hands, gave it Reiki and treated it for ten minutes with my breath. As I did this I wrote a power symbol with my tongue and then blew this on its trembling little body. The next day we were already watching this duckling make its first attempts to swim.

Aura Massage with Reiki

Prerequisite:
1ˢᵗ Reiki Degree

Technical Instructions

Step 1: Have the client lie on her back. Sit next to her at the level of the stomach.

Step 2: Place one hand on your own 6ᵗʰ chakra (forehead) and the other hand on your own 4ᵗʰ chakra (heart). After about a minute ask your Inner Child to help heal the client's aura with a massage healing. If there is a specific problem you can also pray for its healing.

Step 3: After another minute in the same position hold your arms above the client's stomach or heart area so that your lower arms are positioned at about a 90° angle to the upper arms. The palms of your hands are facing the client's body. The distance between both hands is about 30 centimeters (12 inches). Spread your fingers very slightly.

Hold your arms and hands in this position during the entire treatment (90° angle between upper and lower arm and palms of the hands facing the client's body).

Step 4: Now relax the muscles in the upper arms and shoulders as much as possible. The movement required for the aura massage occurs solely through the shoulder joints. Just how relaxed you are can be determined by having someone gently push your arms. If they swing back and forth without any resistance they are relaxed.

In this state most people's arms will begin to move on their own in various patterns which are guided by the Inner Child from the subconscious mind. The movement should never be produced consciously! This is a matter of allowing the Inner Child, the body consciousness, to take charge of the aura massage.

Follow the movements of your arms. Allow any type of movement: circular, elliptical and linear movements, even movements from top to bottom. If the arms want to move more toward the legs or the head then your body must, of course, follow as well.

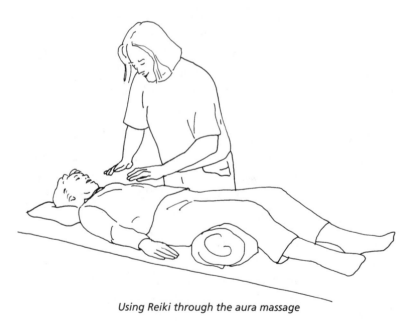

Using Reiki through the aura massage

The aura massage reaches its natural end when the movement of the arms comes to a standstill. Always wait for about 30 seconds once the arms have ceased moving. Experience has shown that the movement may begin again after a short break. If the treatment has to be ended prematurely for some reason say: "Dear Inner Child please end the aura massage now in the most healing way possible for the client." The movement of your arms will then quickly come to rest when the Inner Child has taken the necessary measures. In no case should you simply remove your arms from the client's body without addressing the energy!

If you have been initiated into the 2nd Degree Reiki you can establish a distance contact with the Inner Child rather than treating the 4th and 6th charkas. In this case maintain the connection until the end of the treatment. At the beginning ask the Inner Child for its cooperation in the aura massage and increase the flow of the Reiki force by invoking several intensification signs. In conclusion thank the Inner Child before leaving the distance contact.

Length
At least 5 minutes. The exact treatment time depends upon the individual problems.

Please Note
The length of aura massages differs greatly since the Inner Child adapts itself precisely to the individual needs in each situation. The free intuitively guided movement detailed above and the position of the arms and hands are decisive for the healing effect of the aura massage.

Should there be difficulties with the independent movement of the arms the following program is often helpful in building a good relationship with the Inner Child and developing a
healthy ability to resonate.

Drink a good amount of fresh water every day,
which means at least 35 ml per kilogram of body
weight every day. Avoid eating meat or meat
products. Eliminate sugar and white flour as well
as alcohol and other drugs from your life. At least
one-third of your overall daily diet should con-
sist of fresh fruit and vegetables (organically
grown if possible—it makes a huge difference!).
Take a good supplement of vital elements such
as vitamins, minerals, trace elements and en-
zymes. Walk for at least half an hour every day
and give yourself a daily half-hour massage. In
addition be sure that there is more and more
cheerfulness and laughter in your life every day.

Use

Every type of physical, emotional, mental or spiritual disharmony.

Combination

In principle the aura massage is a complete treatment method in itself. In many cases it can be
made even more effective by combining it with
other techniques. In my practice I often use it
together with the following applications: Contacting the angels or the power animals, mental
healing, KarmaClearing, crystal healing, Reiki for
the Inner Child.

Philosophy

The Inner Child (body consciousness) directly
perceives the energies of living beings and has a
broad spectrum of abilities for healing energy

work. The conscious mind (middle self) can indirectly perceive energies and perform energy work only through the Inner Child. With the aura massage the Inner Child is given the space to use its talents independently for healing and harmonization. This is very effective. If the aura massage is done regularly healing power quickly increases and the ability to perceive energies becomes intensified.

What Works? What Doesn't?

Any type of disharmony as explained above can be treated in this way. If there is an acute physical problem like a broken bone or a cut this should be treated additionally by laying hands on the damaged area. If it is necessary to harmonize addictions, compulsive behavior, fears or fixations, mental healing and systematic chakra work are useful.

All of these measures practiced within the scope of the home and family healing arts should be used only as a complement to treatment provided by a medical professional.

Experiences A Reiki friend frequently uses the aura massage to treat her pets, a dog and two cats. The animals respond very well and greatly prefer such treatments to contact treatments. The cats always start purring immediately the treatment starts.

Aura—Sweeping Down with Reiki

Prerequisite:

1ˢᵗ Reiki Degree

Technical Instructions

before a Reiki Treatment.

Step 1: Wash your hands and rinse your mouth.

Step 2: With both hands slowly sweep down the client's entire body at a distance of about 10 to 20 centimeters (4 to 8 inches). Start about 10 to 20 centimeters above the head and continue to about 10 to 20 centimeters below the feet.

The client can be lying down, sitting or standing while you do this.

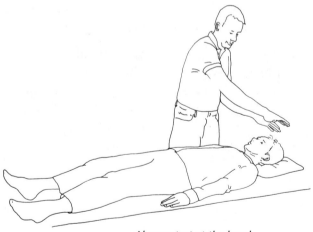

Always start at the head

It doesn't matter whether you sweep down the front or back of the body. You can either sweep your hands above the middle of the body or along the sides, both together.

If you would like to intensify the effect even more and have been initiated into the 2nd Reiki Degree then visualize the power symbol physically strengthening your client. Use the mental-healing symbol followed by the power symbol to support him on the mental and emotional levels. As usual every symbol should be drawn once, if only in your mind, and its Mantra repeated three times silently.

Length   10 to 20 seconds.

Please Note   This technique has two parts. The first part is done before the treatment, the second after the treatment (see the following technique of Aura—Sweeping Up, page 76).

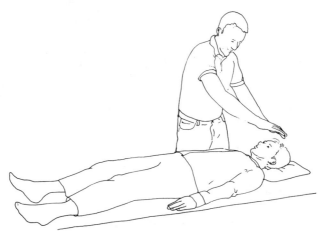

Hold your hands about 10-20 cm (4-8 inches) away from the body

73

Use   This technique is always used before a treatment to help the client's body absorb Reiki energy during the treatment.

Combination This technique is used before every treatment in order to prepare the energy of the client.
Whole-body treatment, distant healing treatment and deprogramming.

Philosophy   The aura is like a blackboard upon which specific instructions are written for the individual. Before a treatment we use this technique to wipe away all of the prevailing instructions so that we can treat the body exactly as it would like to be treated beyond its energetic patterns.

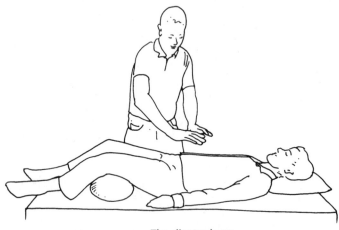

The client relaxes

With this technique we can create a good platform for a treatment but energetic patterns can only be temporarily suspended this way. For a far-reaching aura treatment refer to the Aura Massage on page 67.

Experiences   Our clients report that they feel as if they are wrapped in a warm, light and bright protective shield through this quick aura work.

I once used this technique very slowly and carefully on a ten-year-old girl. The little girl sat on a chair and fell into a deep sleep within 20 seconds! So whenever you want to help someone fall asleep or calm someone down ....

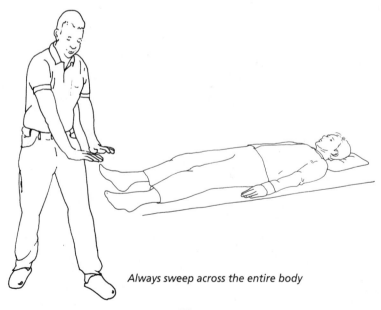

Always sweep across the entire body

Aura—Sweeping Up with Reiki

Prerequisite:
1st Reiki Degree

Technical Instructions
Use this after a Reiki treatment.

With both hands make a single strong sweep up the aura at a distance of about 10 to 20 centimeters (4 to 8 inches) from the client's body starting at her *Dantien* (two to three fingerwidths beneath the navel). Stop at about 10 to 20 centimeters above the head.

Time   3 to 5 seconds.

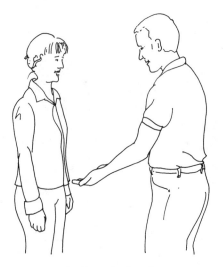

Begin at the Dantien ...

Please Note	This technique has two parts. The first part is done before the treatment, the second after the treatment. (See the technique of Aura—Sweeping Down on pages 72-75.)
Use	This technique is always used after a treatment to help the body refrain from falling directly back into its old patterns.
Combination	Whole-body treatment, distant healing treatment, deprogramming.
Philosophy	The aura has a number of tasks. For one it provides us with a protective shield. It is also an information carrier. If we have worked on the physical as well as on the mental and emotional bodies it is important to harmonize the aura at the end of the treatment so that it is capable of accommodating the 'new' energy.

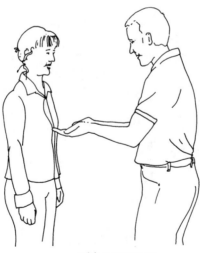

with momentum

77

What Works? What Doesn't?

This technique is designed to help the treatment develop lasting effects. However every body has its own specific habits and it is not capable of breaking all of these. Yes, the state of balance after the treatment will at least last somewhat longer.

Experiences   After a Reiki treatment the client is often a little dazed. This technique will wake up the client and simultaneously allow her go back to everyday life in a refreshed state of mind.

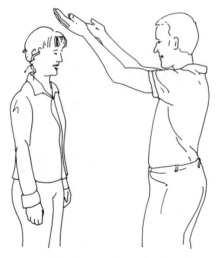

4 to 8 inches above the head

Bath Water—Charging with Reiki

Prerequisite:

2nd Reiki Degree

Technical Instructions

Step 1: Hold your hands above the bath water.

Step 2: Draw the mental-healing symbol once and mentally repeat the Mantra three times.

Step 3: Seal everything with the power symbol (draw it once, repeat the Mantra three times).

Step 4: Let the energy flow ....

Step 5: In addition run your hand through the bath water several times to distribute the energy throughout the entire tub.

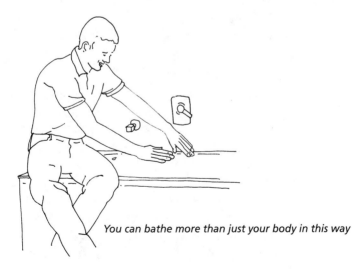

You can bathe more than just your body in this way

Length	2 Minutes.
Please Note	In many cultures baths are used as spiritual rituals. Without much effort when we bathe we can imagine washing off not only the dirt and sweat of everyday life but also our worries and whatever is clinging to us from the past.
Use	This technique can help you enrich the bath water with Reiki energy and allows you be treated by it after a long day.
Combination	Distant healing treatment, distant healing treatment of situations in the future or past.
Philosophy	Water absorbs information and energy like no other element. Only the human body exceeds water in its ability to conduct Reiki energy. We can take advantage of this knowledge by using a technique.

Not only will drinking Reiki charged water help us to better health and more vitality but bathing in it will also do the trick. Proximity to a murmuring stream, a waterfall or even a fountain charges us with energy. We can intensify this also by enriching the water in the area where we live with Reiki.

What Works? What Doesn't?

This technique, like many of the other methods described in this book is intended to provide our body with additional energy. However we must also look after our body, take care of it and love it as our best friend. When we are completely drained we have mistreated our body-mind. We should avoid doing this. Let's be kind to ourselves!

Experiences   Over the years I have grown accustomed to many good things in my host country, Japan. One Japanese ritual that has grown dear to my heart is taking a hot bath in the evening. I enrich the bath water with Reiki using the Reiki symbols of either the 2nd or the 3rd Degrees as described above. Or I simply sit in the bathtub and let the energy flow into the water from all the cells of my body. In this way what is within flows out and what is on the outside flows back in again. The cycle is complete.

Bodywork and Reiki

Prerequisite:

1st Reiki Degree

For anyone who practices Reiki, the healing and personality development method that originated in Japan, it is obvious that spiritual life energy reaches the body through the touch of the hands. Via sequences of positions which vary from school to school, the organism is relaxed and its life functions, its metabolism, its diet, detoxification, purification and the regeneration of cells are all stimulated with Reiki.

In this process the positions of the hands are usually either prescribed by a set treatment plan or they are found intuitively through subtle perception. In addition to laying on of hands during Reiki sessions helpful complementary bodywork is usually only done by trained professionals. I think this is quite unfortunate since non-professionals can also give easily applied and very effective types of bodywork that increase the beneficial effects of Reiki. This boosts the body's receptivity to the universal life energy and improves the flow after dissolving blocks.

So I would like to pass on to you some of my 'secrets' in this section and give you some tips from my own work.

Technical Instructions

Finding and Pampering Harmony Zones

In addition to the erogenous zones of which everyone is certainly aware, the human being has regions on the body that sometimes like to be held firmly and which respond to such attention with an increased sense of well-being.

There are various approaches explaining this, from the recently developed science of psycho-neuroimmunology to Traditional Chinese Medicine and Indian Tantra. The important thing is that wonderful results occur as a result of touching these zones. It matters little whether it is the nerve reflex zones that increase the production of endorphins in the brain, the acupuncture meridians that are normalized in their function through the transfer of energy or the chakras and nadis that are stimulated by touch. The experts can rack their brains about this while the more practically oriented amongst us allow themselves to be pampered!

Just how exactly does Reiki relate to these harmony zones? The first thing we do is take inventory to determine exactly which regions of the body are the harmony zones. Anyone who is very aware of the body knows them and can probably list some of them. Otherwise the easiest way to find them is through experimenting.

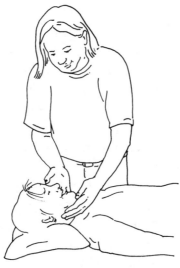

Reiki for well-being

In my experience many people have these zones in the area of the waist, the upper arms, the back and side parts of the throat as well as on the hands and feet.

Test these regions on your client by calmly placing your hands on them and hold them quite firmly. This however really must be pleasant for the client! After only a short time, maybe 20 to 30 seconds, he can usually say if the touch feels especially good. Since the harmony zones are not necessarily very large (many have the diameter of a saucer, some are only as large as a silver dollar), it is important to look for them and try them out several times. After a little experience it often becomes increasingly easy for the client to say exactly where the hands should be placed once they are close to a harmony zone.

It is helpful to draw those harmony zones which have been found on a sketch of the human body showing both the front and the back. The next session can then get started right away without any major preparation. By consulting related literature you will be able to draw some interesting conclusions about the meridians, acupuncture points, reflex zones, chakras and the like.

You will quickly discover that an understanding of harmony zones adds extraordinarily valuable dimensions to the effectiveness of Reiki. After all, the body attracts universal life energy, especially when it experiences the associated touch as enjoyable and pleasant. The harmony zones are actually a type of open door to the body which loves be touched and held.

I have often noticed that treating the harmony zones also causes other areas of the body to become more sensitive to the Reiki energy. In the course of several sessions more or less distinct harmony zones develop in these areas as well. Furthermore the body consciousness of the client grows in leaps and bounds from treatment to treatment and his attitude toward his own body becomes more harmonious and loving.

Whether or not the client is dressed is of no consequence in this form of treatment. I personally find it more sensible to treat a person dressed unless they are your own partner, or the practitioner and client are used to bodywork and can approach it in a balanced way. In any case this needs to be discussed with the client before a Reiki treatment involving harmony zones.

Speaking of the partner, giving each other hours of pampering with Reiki and harmony-zone treatments can bring a great deal of tenderness and loving intimacy into a relationship. This way both people can get to know each other better and treat one another with more sensitivity.

Ways to Increase the Body's Receptivity to Reiki

When Reiki simply does not want to flow, even though it is needed for such problems as stomachaches or coughs, a few bodywork tricks can be very helpful. The techniques described here are anyway very effective for intensifying the flow of Reiki. Even Reiki 1st Degree practitioners can be use them safely and simply to increase the effect of the treatments and more quickly restore harmony.

Blowing On a Person

Since the beginning of time blowing breath onto a person has been an important part of spiritual healing rituals. It can be used to unlock blocked regions of the body that do not want to accept Reiki, or to increase the intensity of a treatment.

When you do this it is important to ask the creative force for its assistance in the healing. Imagine drawing in with your breath the golden healing light that flows to you from the heavens.

Gather it in the region of the *hara,* a point about two finger-widths below the navel. Now exhale the healing spiritual energy and blow it onto the area of the body that you are treating. Repeat this process three times and after each breath wait for half to one minute so that it can have its full effect. Then lay on your hands as usual. Reiki will now flow much better than before.

Anyone who has been initiated into the 2nd Reiki Degree can strengthen the effect of this technique by using the tongue to draw the power symbol and then using the corresponding Mantra to blow the sign onto the area of the body being treated.

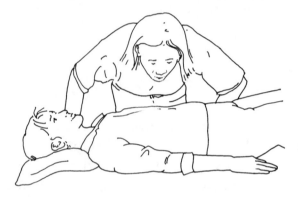

Dissolving Blocks in the Joints

Blocks can easily collect in and around the joints disrupting the free flow of energies in the body. While on the one hand this may mean that Reiki will not be absorbed well, on the other, energies releasing from blocks which Reiki is dissolving are held back. They want to move out of the body through the hands and feet but cannot.

In order to dissolve extensive blocks in the joints proceed in the following manner: First ask your client to move the joint in question gently and very slowly back and forth a number of times. This should be done like slow motion. After this little exercise simply place your hands on it and let Reiki flow. You can also use the technique of blowing on it or the Homeopathic Touch with Reiki (see page 168).

When you work on these joints regularly the organism will experience an overall increase in sensitivity and flexibility. As a result it will also have a much stronger response to healing energetic stimuli such as Reiki, Bach Flowers, homeopathy, shiatsu, herbal naturopathy or healing stones, and can better help improve its own health.

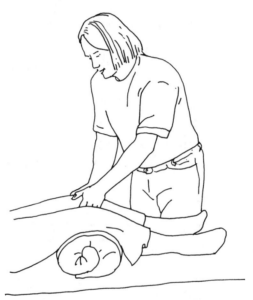

A pillow or rolled-up blanket under the knees promotes relaxation

Length   Depends on the state of the client's health. This must be tested in individual cases until the energy flows.

Please Note   *During a Reiki sessions it is imperative to consider that a person may be afraid of this much intimacy.* Not everyone is accustomed to being touched all over the body. Many people become fearful when they are subjected to touch for the long periods which are routine and necessary for Reiki treatments. It is very important to pay attention to this.

A good approach toward a client new to Reiki sessions is to take time to talk in order for him or her to 'warm up'. Explain the process and ask them whether they may be feeling nervous about the treatment. This helps creates trust and will effectively underpin a good relationship between client and practitioner.

If there are major fears about touching in the initial sessions Reiki can be given exclusively through the feet or hands. These areas have an extraordinary number of reflex zones through which the spiritual life energy can reach the entire body. In addition this is an opportunity to locate the harmony zones.

In dealing with fears related to touch and closeness it is especially important to encourage the client to give feedback often so that the practitioner understands the degree of enjoyment engendered by this type of touch.

Use Creating receptivity for Reiki and other naturopathic treatments, strengthening the flow of energy, dissolving blocks in the body, supporting flexibility, integrating feelings of dislocation.

Combination Among others, whole-body treatment, special positions, chakra balancing.

Philosophy   According to the Arndt-Schulze Law (see page 169) gentle stimuli arouse vital energy and strong stimuli obstruct it. The techniques explained above use this law in reintegrating areas of the body that no longer participate fully in its energy metabolism. This helps such areas back into the natural order of the body's own energy system.

What Works? What Doesn't?

Receptivity to healing influences can be increased very effectively. In some cases actual healing may even take place. However, restorative treatments are usually necessary to completely re-establish harmony.

Experiences   In my experience being aware of bodywork therapy during Reiki sessions can be especially helpful. It can create healing impulses for psychological problems and assist the body in freeing itself from stubborn blocks. Imbalances in the way the spine and the joints are related to each other are also better corrected in this way.

Candle Ritual with Rainbow Reiki

Prerequisite:

2nd Reiki Degree

Technical Instructions

Step 1: Take three candles, white or violet in color. Candles made of bees wax are very good for this purpose. The candles should not contain any artificial fragrance. In addition you need about two handfuls of white quartz sand and a plate on which to put the candle later plus a piece of paper and a pen.

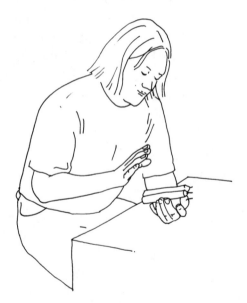

Charging candles with spiritual power

Step 2: Place the candle, the paper, the pen, the plate and the sand under a strong Reiki shower for 24 hours in a room that has been treated with the Rainbow Reiki room-cleansing technique.

Step 3: Taking one at a time roll each candle back and forth between your hands until the surface has become somewhat soft. Hold your hands in warm water for a moment before you roll the candle and the wax will become soft more quickly.

Step 4: Shake some of the sand onto a white piece of paper and roll each candle on it applying slight pressure until the entire surface is covered with sand pressed into the wax.

Step 5: Give the candle a mental treatment for about 10 minutes, add a positive affirmation or positive wish for the person to be treated.

Step 6: Fix the candles onto the plate so that they form an equilateral triangle.

Step 7: Place the piece of paper containing a positive request for the client in the center of the candles. Be sure that the person's name and date of birth are included. Optimally a photo or a sample of the client's handwriting is included.

Step 8: Hold each of the candles for a moment. Ask the creative force to bless what you are doing and that it may benefit everyone.

Step 9: Light each of the candles. While lighting the first say: "Truth!" Lighting the second say: "Love!" And the third say: "Personal responsibility!"

Step 10: Build a strong Reiki shower above the candles and let them burn for at least five minutes. 15 minutes would be even better.

Step 11: If you are working on a larger project that requires more time renew the Reiki shower every day. Burn the candles every day and exchange the used ones for new candles that have been prepared in the same manner.

Step 12: If you want to end the ritual do not put the candles and the paper in the trash but bury them in the ground giving thanks and creating a Reiki shower on this spot.

Length

This technique can be used for a few hours or longer periods up to several weeks or even months. How long you use it depends on how long the desired healing or growth process calls for.

Please Note

This technique should only be used with the explicit consent of the person to be treated. Requests must always be formulated in a positive way. The Rainbow Reiki candle ritual also makes it possible to provide groups, planet Earth, power spots, towns, forests and countries with harmonizing spiritual energy.

Use

Among other things a profound constructive influence and the reshaping of a disharmonious life, environmental and personality structures, support in the healing of serious illnesses, to dissolve major healing blocks, fears, depressions, hopelessness and harmful habits.

Combination Among other things KarmaClearing, distant healing treatment, Reiki for the Inner Child, Reiki for the Higher Self, Rainbow Reiki light-bodywork, mental healing, systematic chakra work.

Philosophy The candles symbolize the transformation of material structures into spiritual forces. Through the quartz sand* we can program them with the appropriate Rainbow Reiki techniques for healing and promote personal development which at this intensity would usually only be possible using crystals.

Since Reiki, the spiritual life energy, is the mediating, activating and connecting factor here, this technique cannot be misused. No information that is hostile to life can be sent through the Reiki channel. Because of the space-holder at the center and the good intentions written on the paper, positive and spiritual influences will reach the person who has been named.

What Works? What Doesn't?

Depending on the strength of the resistance in the way of a positive development some cases require additional energy work techniques, as well as illuminating and inspiring counseling.

Experiences Through a case of mistaken identity the son of one of my Reiki students was jailed in Thailand. She was very afraid for him and asked me whether she might somehow help him with Rainbow Reiki. I advised her to do the Rainbow Reiki candle ritual.

---

* Quartz sand is quartz crystal that has been extremely fine ground.

93

Although she had never done anything like this before she was ready to try it. Three days after she started the ritual for her son the error was clarified and he was released.

Chakras—Opening and Closing with Reiki

Prerequisite:

1st Reiki Degree

Technical Instructions

> *Step 1:* Hold one hand above the relevant energy center for a while and feel into it. Focus your attention on it.

> *Step 2:* Move your hand slowly and gently in three counterclockwise circles above the chakra. Ask that the chakra open itself and visualize a flower

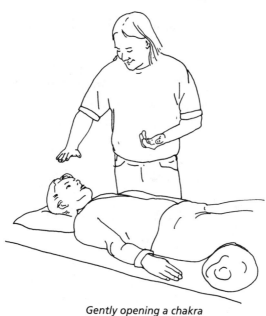

Gently opening a chakra

95

opening as you do this. Feel the change in the way the chakra radiates.

Step 3: Now treat the chakra with the cloud hands. To do this move your hands gently back and forth as if they are dancing in the wind. Allow 'It' to move your hands so that the control of the movement occurs spontaneously. You can also use the power symbol, the Reiki power ball or a healing gemstone that you have carefully cleansed and activated beforehand. Or you can sing the power song "Hey loa, key loa", or vowels, etc.

Step 4: To close a chakra attune yourself again as described above. Then move your hand gently and calmly above it three times in clockwise circles. As you do this visualize a flower closing.

Step 5: In conclusion let Reiki flow into the energy center a little longer. When you are done you may want to apply the grounding technique, chakra balancing or give the Inner Child Reiki (through distance contact).
Rest is recommended afterward.

Length   About 3 to 10 minutes.

Please Note   Always approach an open chakra in a very sensitive and careful way. Never forget to close an opened chakra when the work has been done.

Use   To exert healing influence on a deep-rooted imbalance within a chakra, to clear and heal blocked chakras, to work purposefully on specific energetic structures within a chakra.

Combination   Systematic chakra work, chakra balancing, crystal treatment of a chakra.

Philosophy   By opening a chakra its receptivity for healing energies is extensively increased.

What Works? What Doesn't?

A chakra can be very intensely influenced for healing.

However the formation of new, healthy structures within a chakra sometimes requires many months. Such treatment must be complemented by counseling and decisions in favor of a harmonious lifestyle in areas affected by the chakra in question. It is possible that other techniques of energy work and psychotherapy or spiritual consultation may also be needed.

Experiences   A physician who is a friend of mine once asked me to help a cancer patient with Reiki sessions. These were in addition to his own treatment. The illness was already quite advanced and, as frequently occurs in such cases, it was difficult to trigger a healing response. The body had already been subjected to so much stress through the previous chemotherapy and radiation therapies.

Only by specifically opening the afflicted major chakra and secondary chakras was it possible for Reiki to penetrate to the roots of this terrible disease. It took more than a year with many contact and distant healing treatments as well as intensive therapy with homeopathy, vital substances, aloe vera and cat's claw to conquer that cancer.

In retrospect I can say that the turning point toward healing occurred with the beginning of the Reiki treatment on the opened chakras.

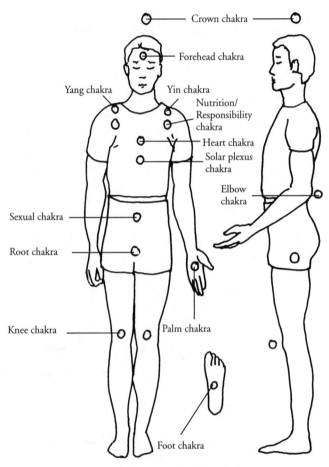

The major and secondary chakras

Comatose Patients—Treating with Reiki

Prerequisite:

2nd Reiki Degree

Technical Instructions

Step 1: Sitting or standing in a relaxed way with your feet parallel to each other, take several deep breaths.

Step 2: Now draw the distance-treatment symbol once in the way that is most comfortable for you and mentally repeat the corresponding Mantra three times.

Step 3: Repeat the name of the client three times.

Step 4: Say: "I am making contact with the consciousness of ... (name of the client)."

Step 5: Draw the mental-healing symbol once and repeat the Mantra three times.

Step 6: Now seal everything with the power symbol (draw it once, say the Mantra three times).

I have often noticed a silent dialog developing between client and practitioner within just a few minutes. This dialog takes place on an intuitive level in the mind.

Mentally ask the client what you can do for him. It is possible that you will be asked to treat specific areas of the body. Follow your intuition and during the treatment pay attention to the client's body language.

An intuitive conversation may develop psychically. It may be that the client is afraid of dying and asks you for instruction in the art of passing on. This type of treatment demands a clear head and the first prerequisite for it is that you are not afraid death yourself.

Another possibility is that your client asks you to help him have the strength and energy to die. You can proceed to do this with a whole-body treatment or, if very little time remains, by treating the *Dantien* (two to three fingerwidths below the navel).

Length   15 to 60 minutes or longer if necessary

Please Note   For the practitioner two things are especially important in this technique. Firstly, your attitude toward life and death and to your client. We do not know what is good for the client. When his time comes death will be the right thing for him and it would be wrong to want to interfere.

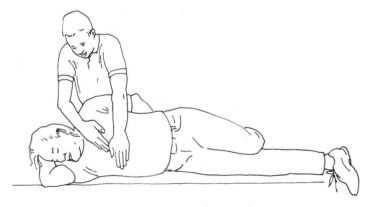

Connected in the silence of existence with Reiki

Secondly, your attitude toward yourself. You cannot and are not permitted to try to take away anyone else's suffering. After the treatment you leave the client where he is and continue your own life. At the close of the treatment mentally say to the client: "And now with love and respect I disassociate myself from your destiny." Afterwards it is helpful for the practitioner to rest.

Use　　In the apparently hopeless situation of a comatose client you can use the Reiki symbols to make contact with their consciousness.

Combination　Reiki treatment with the 1st Degree, Reiki treatment with the 2nd Degree, distance Reiki, affirmation technique (caution: this should only be done after getting the client's approval beforehand if this is possible).

Philosophy　A coma is not what it appears to be. Comatose patients are often conscious at a deeper level. To a certain extent they can perceive what is happening around them. If possible speak with the client out loud and psychically obtain his permission.

This is worth a try: Ask the client if he can hear and watch to see whether an eyelid moves, a finger stretches or there is a change in the breathing rhythm. This may be in response to the question. There have been cases where a patient has shown a tiny signal which through painstaking effort can be developed more and more. If there are other visitors present and such 'craziness' would be out of place this can be done mentally with the help of the 2nd Reiki Degree symbols.

What Works? What Doesn't?

Using this technique we can put an end to the frustration that most of us experience in dealing with comatose patients.

Experiences   An aunt of mine slipped into a coma just before her death. Unlike all her other visitors I would leave the hospital each day at peace with myself, conscious that I had done my best for her. And, as a bonus after every visit for a couple of days, she would wake up out of her depths joking with those around her before sinking back into the coma again .... Nothing in this world is permanent!

Connecting with the Reiki Force

Prerequisite:
1ˢᵗ Reiki Degree

2ⁿᵈ Reiki Degree for Variation 5

Technical Instructions
This technique has several variations. Experiment with it and you will see which form has the best results for you.

Variation 1   *Step 1:* Sit or stand comfortably and take a few deep breaths.

Step 2: Fold your hands with your palms together and slowly raise them until they are above your crown chakra with the fingertips pointing to the sky.

Step 3: Wait until you feel a tingling in the fingertips and the hand chakras. In a minute or two you will probably feel the energy entering your crown chakra. This may be felt as warmth, light, a tingling or a magnetic feeling.

Step 4: Now spread the Reiki energy in your aura with both hands.

Step 5: Begin with the treatment or self-treatment.

Variation 2   *Step 1:* Sit or stand comfortably and take a few deep breaths.

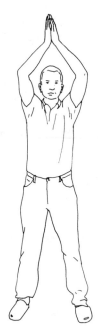

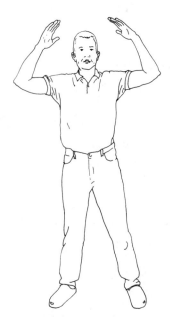

Attune yourself to the Reiki energy   *Spread the energy in your aura*

Step 2: Fold your hands in front of your heart and ask the Reiki energy to flow through you. You will now begin to feel the energy in your crown chakra, your heart chakra or in your hands and feet.

Step 3: Begin with the treatment or self-treatment.

Variation 3   *Step 1:* Sit or stand comfortably and take a few deep breaths.

Step 2: Ask the Reiki energy to flow through you.

Step 3: Now rub your hands together a few times very vigorously to warm them and activate your hand chakras.

Step 4: Open your hands with the little fingers still touching and blow into them once with the intention of activating your hands.

Step 5: Begin with the treatment or self-treatment.

Variation 4   *Step 1:* Sit or stand comfortably and take a few deep breaths.

Step 2: In your mind say: "The Reiki energy is flowing."

Step 3: Begin with the treatment or self-treatment.

Variation 5   *Step 1:* Sit or stand comfortably and take a few deep breaths.

Step 2: Draw the distance-treatment symbol once and mentally repeat the corresponding Mantra three times.

Step 3: Then say: "I hereby connect with the Reiki energy." If you want the Reiki energy flow for a specific length of time say: "I ask the Reiki energy to flow from ... to ...."

Step 4: Now draw the mental-healing symbol once and repeat the Mantra three times.

Step 5: Seal everything with the power symbol (draw it once, repeat the Mantra mentally three times).

Step 6: Begin with the treatment or self-treatment.

Length	1 to 3 minutes plus the time of the treatment.
Please Note	It is necessary to rest afterward. You should not drive in traffic or do anything calling for complete concentration during or shortly after the treatment. Afterwards take at least 15 minutes before you re-immerse yourself in the 'seriousness of life.'
Use	We can connect with the Reiki energy before we give a treatment or when we want to charge ourselves with energy with the help of this technique.
Combination	Whole-body treatment, Reiki distant healing treatment, affirmation technique.
Philosophy	Many of us do not need a technique to feel the flow of Reiki energy. We also don't need to turn the energy on or off. It flows always and everywhere whether we are asleep or awake. With this technique we simply awaken our consciousness to it.

What Works? What Doesn't?

This technique cannot make us fit when we have exhausted ourselves even if it does connect us with Reiki energy.

When a new Reiki student came to us a few years ago I was very surprised at her condition. Although she already had the 3rd Reiki Degree she was both physically and psychically run down.

I thought privately that someone practicing Reiki could never become so worn out. It turned out that her Reiki teacher had told her to go on giving Reiki treatments especially if she felt sick and weak and that the energy flowing through

106

both the practitioner and the recipient would get her moving again.

Although in theory this may be right, the top priority is for us to recover whenever we are ill or somehow physically weakened. The first rule of Reiki is: Be good to yourself.

Go to bed when you are sick!

Experiences At almost every one of my seminars I am asked the best way to 'turn on' the energy. My standard answer is always: "Go ahead and try to turn it off!"

Crystal Fountains with Rainbow Reiki

Prerequisite:
2nd Reiki Degree

Technical Instructions

Step 1: Activate three pieces of rose quartz, three amethysts, and three quartz crystals,* all about the size of a walnut as explained in the exercise, 'Healing Stones—Activating with Rainbow Reiki' (see page 164).

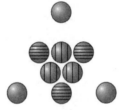

Order of the healing stones for the Rainbow Reiki crystal fountains

Key:
- RQ = rose quartz
- AM = amethyst
- QC = quartz crystal

---

* In place of the amethysts you can also use fluorite, citrine, smoky quartz or rubies. In place of the rose quartz you can use rhodochrosite, thulite, carnelian or moss agate. Do not substitute anything for the quartz crystals because they bring a considerable increase in the vibrations of the field, aid cleansing of the room energies and the charging of spiritual light energies. If however you use Herkimer diamonds rather than regular quartz crystals the effect of the Rainbow Reiki crystal fountains will be increased even more.

Step 2: Lay out the stones as depicted in the above illustration.

Step 3: Create a strong Reiki shower above the Rainbow Reiki crystal layout patterns.

Step 4: Every 3 to 10 days create a new Reiki shower and thank the crystals and the angels who work through them for their help.

Length

The pattern is intended for constant use. If you would like to remove it please thank the crystals and the angels that work through them for their support.

Please Note

Since a positive influence can also be an invasion of privacy, only build the patterns in the rooms or gardens of other people with their express approval.

If the patterns need to be temporarily removed keep the crystals in a bag that is reserved for them only until they are used again. (The bag should be made of natural materials if possible).

Use

For the general increase of vibrations in homes and gardens. A comprehensive, very strong field of Reiki and high-frequency extremely illuminating crystal energy is achieved when such a pattern is laid at the four corners of an apartment, house or garden as well as at the center of this pattern.

An even more complex and intense field occurs when we lay eight patterns, each precisely in the direction of the eight points of the compass,*

---

* North, south, east, west, northeast, northwest, southeast, and southwest.

plus one at the center of the piece of property, house or apartment.

Render the crystal patterns permanent and transportable like this: Fill a plate or flowerpot saucer of the appropriate size with half to one inch of moist clay and then press the crystals into the clay. You can purchase the clay in any craft or hardware store. As soon as the clay has dried the stones are set. If you wish to use it in outside areas like gardens you should use plaster instead of clay since it is more weatherproof.

Our observations have shown that Rainbow Reiki crystal fountains in gardens gradually bring a distinct improvement to quality of the soil, more harmonious and vital plant growth, a larger variety of species and a tangibly more positive atmosphere.

Rainbow Reiki crystal mandalas can help in the regeneration of forests, bodies of water and landscapes that have been damaged through pollution. In city residences crystal fountains can provide effective protection against radiations rising from technology as well as a stable, powerful natural quality of energy.

Placed by the bed of a patient crystal fountains brighten the mood and improve healing processes and convalescence. They can help the dying take leave of earthly life in a calm and peaceful way.

In meditation and healing rooms as well as in spiritual centers they help increase the vibration so that it becomes easier to distance oneself from everyday life and turn to areas such as personal development, relaxation, meditation, truth and love.

At places of work the atmosphere becomes more relaxed, constructive and creative. And the work gets done more easily.

Pets also like to have a Rainbow Reiki crystal fountain next to their food or where they sleep.

Combination Room cleansing, Reiki shower, contact with the Higher Self or Inner Child of a house or garden, Rainbow Reiki KarmaClearing for buildings and landscapes.

Philosophy Reiki from the Reiki shower encourages the crystals to transmit stronger healing powers. This helps human beings, animals and plants to become not only more whole but also to become receptive to Reiki. Like the alchemical process of *solve et coagula** or the homeopathic dilution, Rainbow Reiki healing-stone activation releases strong spiritual healing powers. This makes the work with crystals much more effective, cleansing is necessary less frequently and the crystals activated in this manner attune themselves more easily to a mutual vibrational field, such as a mandala.

What Works? What Doesn't?

With the Rainbow Reiki crystal fountain strong and pleasant influences can be brought into the material world. According to the type of crystals used other healing energies can be summoned in addition to the powerful Reiki vibration.

---

* Literally: 'dissolve and coagulate'

As with energetic Feng Shui measures, the effects of structural problems may only be diminished in this way. This can have a decisive significance for health, well being and success.

Since the Rainbow Reiki crystal fountain is a very strong instrument for energy work we can expect a great deal from it. Gardens where Rainbow Reiki crystal fountains have been implemented thrive splendidly and their support has made it possible to resolve some of the ongoing struggles.

Influencing factors such as diet, exercise, unhealthy radiation and a great variety of psychological problems can be constructively influenced by using Rainbow Reiki crystal fountains.

This statement also applies in the case of foods, but if there isn't any goodness in it you cannot conjure it up. For mental and emotional problems good counseling, clearing of difficulties, understanding and consciousness work may often be necessary as well to balance greater disharmonies.

Experiences Since we installed several Rainbow Reiki crystal fountains in our garden there are suddenly new species of plants, wild herbs sprouting and lots of bumble-and-other bees and butterflies have appeared. A colony of spotted salamanders has also moved in.

Crystal Healing with Rainbow Reiki

Prerequisite:

1ˢᵗ Reiki Degree

Technical Instructions

Step 1: Select the appropriate healing stones.

Step 2 (optional): Treat them with the Rainbow Reiki healing-stone activation technique (see page 164).

Step 3: Now place the stones on the areas of the body to be treated. If you wish to work on the aura use strips of cotton material about 4 inches wide and 10 to 14 inches long to wrap the crystals and tie them onto your hands so that the stones sit in the center of your palm. Alternatively use thin cotton gloves. Place your hands on the stones and let Reiki take effect.

Step 4: After the end of the session remember to place the healing stones under a strong Reiki shower for several hours. Rinse them off thoroughly under cold running water or lay them on the ground close to the stem of a strong healthy plant.

Length   At least 3 minutes. A more intensive treatment is possible if you correspondingly lengthen the time of the application.

Please Note   The healing stones and crystals are especially effective when they have been treated beforehand with the Rainbow Reiki healing-stone activation (see page 164).

Tumbled quartz crystals (i.e. rounded stones) always do a good job. Specialized stones for particular effects are often used, but quartz is the great mainstay.

If you are attaching the healing stones to your hands it is helpful to place the cotton strips or gloves under a strong Reiki shower over night beforehand. You can also cover them for the same amount of time with a good dozen walnut-sized, tumbled quartz crystals that have been activated with the Rainbow Reiki technique. This will improve their ability to resonate with subtle energies.

Use   Intensification of Reiki treatments, additional influence of healing stone energies, more intensive receptivity of the areas to be treated with Reiki.

Combination   Among others, whole-body treatment, distant healing treatment, special positions, systematic chakra work, chakra balancing, chakra treatment, aura massage, intuitive Reiki.

Philosophy   Reiki stimulates crystals and minerals to transmit stronger and more refined high-frequency healing energies. This is very helpful for treatments. At the same time experience has shown that the energy of the healing stones opens the areas where they are used for Reiki. This means that the spiritual life energy can work more quickly, powerfully and deeply. In turn this supports the response of the organism to the pleasant effects of the healing stones.

Treatment is enormously intensified through the combined influence of Reiki and the powers of healing stones. Moreover additional possibilities for harmonization are activated through the special healing qualities of the individual stones.

However, as also applies to healing work with energies, miracles only occur as the exception to the rule. In order to heal chronic problems most cases require treatment on a regular basis over a considerable period of time.

Experiences One of my Reiki students complained that he felt nothing when he gave himself or others Reiki. He wanted very much to feel spiritual energies in his hands like other people he knew feel them. I recommended that for some time he give treatments of at least 30 minutes using activated quartz crystals. After about 10 days he began to perceive the spiritual healing powers in his hands. He continued doing this for a number of months because he liked the exercise very much and found the new sensations fascinating. Today his hands are so sensitive that he can distinctly detect the fine differences in the energy currents of people's auras.

Deprogramming with Reiki

Prerequisite:

2nd Reiki Degree

Technical Instructions

Before you can begin with deprogramming you need to create an affirmation with the client. This affirmation is to be kept in the present tense. Let it be positive, brief, succinct and expressed in the language of the client. It should not contain any negatively charged words like names of illnesses. In no way should it limit the client.

The creation of an affirmation is an art that should be carried out only by one who knows how the human mind functions.

If possible do not speak with your client during the entire duration of the treatment.

Step 1: Smooth the aura (see pages 72-78: Aura—Sweeping Down/Aura—Sweeping Up).

Step 2: Draw the power symbol on the back of your client's head and mentally repeat the corresponding Mantra three times.

Step 3: Hold the hand you used to draw the symbol above the back of the client's head and let the symbol flow.

Step 4: Draw the mental-healing symbol above the medulla oblongata*. Repeat the Mantra three times and allow the symbol to flow.

---

* Where the spinal cord enters the skull

Step 5: Draw the power symbol above the medulla oblongata and let it flow. Repeat the *Mantra three times allowing it to flow.*

Step 6: Stand next to your client* and place one hand on the back of his head (above the medulla oblongata) and the other hand on his forehead.

Step 7: Imagine that white light is flowing through you from the crown of your head to the soles of your feet. This light now flows through your hands into your client.

Step 8: Repeat the affirmation three times in your mind and feel how it flows through your client.

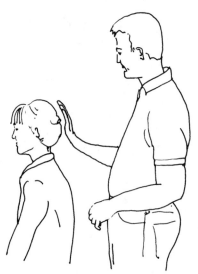

Let the symbols flow

---

* This and the following steps apply if you are working with a client. If you are practicing this technique on yourself they do not apply. Repeat this treatment every day for a week and then twice a week for a longer period. Do not work with more than one affirmation at a time because this scatters the energy.

Step 9: Ask your client to repeat the affirmation silently and as intensely as possible once you have placed one hand on the back of his head and the other on his forehead.

Step 10: Slowly remove your hands from the client's body.

Step 11: Sweep up the aura once (see page 76, Aura—Sweeping Up).

Step 12 (optional): Vigorously rub your hands together five to ten times in order to separate your own energy from the client and the symbols.

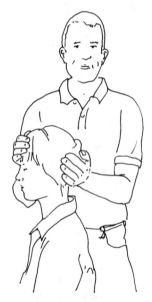

And now the affirmation

Remember to refrain from speaking with your client during the entire treatment if this is possible.

Length	At least 5 to 10 minutes.
Please Note	Rest is necessary afterwards. The client should not drive in traffic right after the session or do any type of work that involves risk or calls for total concentration. Give your client at least fifteen minutes before you allow him back out into the world. A concluding conversation may also be appropriate.
Use	This technique can be used to free a person from undesired habits or to give them new possibilities of action.
Combination	Distant healing treatment, whole-body treatment, karma-cleansing.
Philosophy	Our brain can be compared to the hard drive of a computer. Without software this computer won't work. From early childhood we have all been imprinted and programmed by the people who surround us. With this technique we have the possibility of revoking programming or replacing it with something more desirable. When creating affirmations, which are a form of new programming for the brain, be very careful because once something has been fed in it will stay there, at least until it is changed again.

What Works? What Doesn't?

We cannot convince a person of something that does not fit into his image of the world, his cultural background or conscience and religious beliefs. So we cannot brainwash anyone with an affirmation since the ultimate authority accepting something as true or not is the person himself. This technique is intended to guide the life of the person being treated into more positive channels.

Experiences Using this technique I have successfully convinced myself that life in the 'Here and Now' is the only one worth living. My affirmation for this purpose has been: "I am Here and Now!" After a few months it became increasingly easy for me to live in the present moment. Now this works completely on its own, without the technique.

Distant Healing Treatment in the Future with Rainbow Reiki

Prerequisite:

2nd Reiki Degree

Technical Instructions

Step 1: With the initiated hand draw the distant healing symbol and silently say the corresponding Mantra three times. Then using the same hand draw the power symbol and say the Mantra three times. Visualize the face of the recipient and say their first and last name three times. Immediately imagine written beneath this face the complete date of the day and the time that the Reiki should be received. State the entire date and time three times silently.

Step 2 to Step 9: The procedure is identical with the whole-body treatment in the present moment.

Please Note Be absolutely sure that your client behaves in exactly the same way as for a normal distant healing treatment. In short, sits or lies down comfortably in an available space, certainly not working with any heavy machinery, driving a motor vehicle or doing anything else that requires complete attention. Fifteen minutes of rest is recommended afterwards.

It is of course also possible to do a group distant healing treatment.

Length	Equivalent to a normal distant healing treatment.
Use	You can send yourself or someone else Reiki in advance for future situations when it will be needed at a specific time. It cannot be given directly at that moment because you will be occupied with something else. For example, you would like to be truly free during your vacation but have promised that you will send Reiki to a friend every day. You can do this in a deferred way before your vacation. You will get your peace and quiet and your friend will have his Reiki treatment.
Combination	With any technique that can be used within the scope of a Reiki distant healing treatment.
Philosophy	The Reiki distant healing treatment works through that part of us which exists beyond the everyday time-space continuum. As a result contact can be established with any distant place or individual in both the past and the future.

What Works? What Doesn't?

In general it is more beneficial to provide people with Reiki before examinations, interviews and other important appointments rather than during these critical moments.

Reiki is not a magic trick which can ace any test! However it can be used to help us study better, relax and work through our fears before the big event and for many other purposes along these lines. If you arrive at an examination or interview after a good night's sleep and are well prepared for it, an additional Reiki distant healing treatment can also be a big boost to your situation in the moment.

Experience   I once planned to hold a seminar in Brazil just a few hours after I was to arrive. I wasn't sure that I could overcome the jet lag in such a short time, so during the flight I programmed several distant healing treatments to coincide with the seminar. The event was a complete success. I felt very good and well rested, and had no problems with jet lag at all.

Distant Healing Treatment in the Past with Rainbow Reiki

Prerequisite:

2nd Reiki Degree

Technical Instructions

Step 1: With the initiated hand draw the distance-treatment symbol and quietly say the corresponding Mantra three times. Now use the same hand to draw the power symbol and say or think the Mantra three times. Visualize the face of the recipient and say his first and last name three times. Directly after this visualize the situation to be treated as a still photo, like the flashing of a slide on a screen. It is not important to see the situation exactly as it was. The image should just be appealing to the imagination so that the Inner Child can use it to orient itself.

If you are treating another person have the target situation described as precisely as possible. Imagine that your hands are floating above the situation providing it with Reiki. Naturally you can also use the power-intensification symbol for this purpose.

Step 2: In closing quietly say: "I say goodbye to you ... (add the client's first and last name here) and wish you God's blessing on your way." Blow vigorously between the palms of your hands and then rub them together.

Length	At least 5 minutes. For difficult cases even 30 minutes or longer.
Please Note	This technique can dissolve deep-rooted emotional blocks and make us aware of traumatic experiences. Whole-body treatments, mental healing, Reiki for the Inner Child and Karma-Clearing as well as angel contacts such as with the archangel the divine healer, Raphael, should then be used to facilitate integration or the ultimate release of these undesirables.
Use	When applied regularly Reiki for past situations helps harmonize imbalanced experiences (like birth trauma or the death of friends or relatives) and their effects on the present. Be sure to experiment with this, it's very worthwhile!
	After the treatment the client should have time for himself and express what he has experienced via painting, dancing, sculpting or writing. It is very important to avoid hectic states and stress after the session. Take a cautious approach and first try out this technique on easier cases. Sending Reiki to situations in the past which caused an intense sense of well being is very interesting. The related state will once again be experienced and can help us to relax, mobilize specific energies or overcome times of deep depressions.
Combination	Any technique that can be integrated into a normal Reiki distant healing treatment.
Philosophy	The Reiki distant healing treatment works through that part of a human being existing be-

yond the everyday time-space continuum. As a result contacts can be established with any distant places or individuals in both the past and the future.

What Works? What Doesn't?

The effects of past events can be harmonized and what has occurred can become better integrated into the present. However the past cannot be changed in practical terms. What has happened has happened. We usually do not suffer from what has occurred but from how we understand the experience and include it in our present lives.

Experiences During a consultation a businessman once complained that he always became very fearful when he needed financing for a project. In his childhood his father once suffered great financial difficulties due to excessive debt. From that time on he continuously spoke of loans as evil and dangerous, railing against the banks.

Yet working with credit is important in business because many plans can not be implemented without financing. I recommended that he do the work of treating the past with Rainbow Reiki. After eight weeks of practicing every day with the corresponding situations from his childhood this man approached the negotiation of a large construction project in Spain free from any experience of fear. To this day the problem has not recurred.

Distant Healing Treatment of the Childhood Self

Prerequisite:

2nd Reiki Degree

Technical Instructions

Step 1: Hold a photo of yourself or the person to be treated in your hand.

Step 2: Draw the distance-treatment symbol once on your third eye (or that of your client) and mentally repeat the corresponding Mantra three times.

Step 3: Repeat your name (or that of your client three times) as well as the point in time that is involved. The more precise the point in the past is, the better.

Step 4: Draw the mental-healing symbol once on the heart of the person in the picture and repeat the Mantra three times.

Step 5: Now let the mental-healing symbol flow out of the hand that is suspended above the photo.

Step 6: Stabilize everything with the power symbol (draw it once, repeat the Mantra three times).

Step 7: Place your hands on the photo or hold it in your folded hands (between the palms) as long as you think necessary. If you do not have a photo visualize yourself or your client at the specified time in the past.

Repeat this entire process every day for a week.

Length   10 to 15 minutes.

Please Note This technique brings the past to light and this is not always pleasant. Prepare yourself for tears and pain. If you are working with a client you should always have permission to do this treatment.

It is necessary to rest afterwards. The client should not drive in traffic or do any type of risky work that calls for complete concentration during or shortly after the distant healing treatment. A subsequent conversation on the telephone may be appropriate. If you did not make any notes during the treatment it would be better to speak with your client soon, say within 20 minutes, before you forget what happened during the treatment.

Use   With this technique you can treat conflict situations from your own childhood or that of another person.

Combination Work with the Inner Child, KarmaCleansing, Reiki Box, distant healing treatment, whole-body treatment.

Philosophy Our childhood, especially the first seven years, shape us like no other phase in our life. Little children are vulnerable and receptive to interpretations of their behavior patterns as 'good' or 'bad'. These values become imprinted and reinforced through close contact with other people in the family, at kindergarten, in school etc. Once the brain has been programmed, these patterns become the basis for the way we behave for the rest of our lives. Most people act like small children throughout their entire lifetime!

What Works? What Doesn't?

Even though we have been shaped by the experiences of our childhood, this does not release us from our responsibilities. The moment we have achieved clarity about our past we must learn to let go of it and live in the present moment.

As the old German proverb tells us: "Everyone is the architect of his own fortune (or misfortune)!"

Experiences During the first months working with the 2nd Reiki Degree I used this technique every day. I had the feeling that there were many things I needed to work through.

Firstly I sent Reiki to the traumatic situations in my youth: a hospital stay, difficult times at school and the suicide of a girlfriend. Within a few weeks I had treated the most obvious difficult situations but more and more doors to the past began opening. I remembered things that I had done and experienced in my earliest childhood and spent many hours at night crying on the sofa in my living room.

Fortunately this did not last forever. After about three months I was overcome by feelings of gratitude for everything I have been allowed to experience in my life. From that moment on the details of a life situation no longer play a role for me. I take life as it comes, whether it rains or the sun is shining.

Distant Healing Treatment with a Group

Prerequisite:

2nd Reiki Degree

Technical Instructions

Step 1: On a piece of paper write the first and last names of the people you would like to treat small enough that you can cover all the words with both hands.

Step 2: Draw a distance-treatment symbol above them (the direction does not matter here) and quietly say or think the corresponding Mantra three times in order to activate it.

Step 3: Above all the names draw a large horizontal power symbol and say the Mantra three times.

Step 4: Quietly say each of the first and last names on the paper three times and briefly visualize the face of each person as you do so.

Step 5: Use additional power symbols by drawing them horizontally above the list of names and activate each one with its Mantra in order to intensify the Reiki flow. Place your hands above the names and treat them for about 15 minutes with Reiki. Do it for longer if you have more time.

Step 6 (optional): If you would like to do a mental treatment proceed in the following manner:

Imagine a doll that represents all of the people to be treated and give its head a mental healing meant for the entire group. (This needs to be done first.) Draw the Mental Healing symbol and repeat the Mantra three times. This is followed by the Power symbol plus its Mantra, also three times. (Only after symbols and Mantras are done is the client addressed.) Remember to say quietly the first and last names of each person three times.

Step 7: The group distant healing treatment with Reiki is ended by taking leave of each of your clients by name and then blessing all of them together in the name of the creative force. Then blow vigorously between your hands and rub the palms of your hands together.

Length   At least 10 minutes with no upward time limit.

Please Note   Individual treatments cannot be replaced by the group distant healing treatment. Remember to inform the participants about the time of the distant healing treatment so they do not suddenly find themselves in deep spontaneous relaxation in the middle of the freeway.

Use   Group distant healing treatment of people, as well as animals, plants, buildings and others things can provide them with Reiki through the distance contact. If you have many clients and little time this technique is very helpful in working effectively and at the same time gaining free time for necessary individual consultations and energy-work. It's also a wonderful idea for a group to decide on a regular time for everyone to give one another a group distant healing treatment. The connection among the members becomes closer and many positive effects in personality development and health can occur through this strong energy work. I like to include the planet Earth regularly in-group distant healing treatment.

Combination   Mental healing without a specific focus, Reiki for the Inner Child, Reiki for the Higher Self, distant healing treatment in the future.

Philosophy   Since we can overcome time and space as well as individual differences with the distance-treatment symbol we can provide more than one person at a time with distant healing treatment.

What Works? What Doesn't?

The group distant healing treatment should not be the method you practice the most. You can develop your abilities in the application of Reiki and in subtle perception better through individual treatments. For serious illnesses there are also various reasons for preferring individual treatments. However the group distant healing treatment is always good when you have many clients that need to be provided with Reiki and no time for anything else.

Don't forget to include your own name on every list as well.

Experiences   In seminars I like to use the group distant healing treatment during guided meditations. This allows the participants to open up more to the spiritual world. As a result relaxation occurs more quickly and the reactions to healing through angels and others light beings are much more intense.

Distant Healing Treatment with Rainbow Reiki

Prerequisite:

2nd Reiki Degree

Technical Instructions

Step 1: With the initiated or more skilled hand draw the distance-treatment symbol and silently say the corresponding Mantra three times. Then draw the power symbol with the same hand and silently say the Mantra three times. Visualize the face of the recipient and say their first and last name three times. If you have difficulty imagining the face of the recipient place a photo where you can see it and glance at it now and then so you can remember what they look like.

Step 2: Hold your hands in front of you while imagining that you are treating the face of the recipient. This is the same as in the 1st position of the contact whole-body treatment, to the right and left of the nose from the forehead to the mouth. To intensify this effect you can draw one or more power symbols on the entire face. Remember to activate each symbol by saying the Mantra three times.

Hold your hands in front of you while visualizing that you are treating the ears of the recipient, as in the 3rd position of the whole-body treatment. In all of the places that you are treating use the power symbols and the Mantras to intensify the effect.

Step 3 (Mental healing—optional): Place your uninitiated, less mechanically skilled hand beneath the back of your client's head on the medulla oblongata. With the initiated hand draw a mental-healing symbol on the crown of the head and silently say the Mantra three times. At the same point draw a power symbol and say the Mantra three times. Silently say the recipient's first and last names three times. Use the power symbol and the Mantra several times on the crown of the head to intensify the effect.

Hold your hands in this position until the end of the mental treatment. When you have selected an affirmation for the mental healing repeat it constantly in your mind until you move to the next position.

Step 4: Visualize the entire body of your client in miniature with the face in front of you, the head up and the feet down. Hold your hands to the right and left of the recipient with the palms facing in. Imagine the person so small that your hands can give Reiki from top to bottom without having to change position.

Step 5: Attach the power symbols where you know or intuit that Reiki is especially needed and activate each of them with the corresponding Mantra.

Step 6: Visualize your client's body in such a way that the soles of the feet point toward you. Attach at least one large power symbol to each of them and activate each sign with the Mantra. Grounding is also strengthened through the distant healing treatment just as for the closing position for the whole-body treatment of the 1ˢᵗ Degree. For greater problems with grounding you can also treat the sacrum. Remember that blocked ankles and knees can severely impede the flow of energy from the trunk to the feet obviously also affecting grounding. Treat these areas of the body with Reiki before you work with the soles of the feet.

Step 7: Say silently : "I take leave of you ... (insert your client's first and last name) and wish you the blessing of the creative force (or light and love) on your path."

Step 8: Blow vigorously between the palms of your hands and then rub them together.

For advanced practitioners: All of the steps of the distant healing treatment can of course also be carried out purely on the mental level. But don't begin this too soon so you become truly secure in the technique and can discover errors in the process more easily.

Length   Plan at least 3 minutes of treatment time for each position. Of course there is also no harm in holding them longer. It is often worthwhile giving this treatment for some extra minutes, especially for steps 5 and 6.

Please Note   During and shortly after the distant healing treatment the client should not operate any heavy machines, drive a car or do anything else for which full attention is required.

For operations and anything in which anesthesia or medicinal numbing (dentist!) are necessary remember that Reiki can also help substantially improve the body's ability to detoxify. Reiki can also help harmonize the vasoconstrictive effects of partial anesthesia.

Always remember to say goodbye as in the distant healing treatment which is explained in Step 7.

Use   Reiki applications of all types over a distance, distance perception, distance communication.

Combination Among other things with mental healing, power intensification, chakra work, KarmaClearing, Reiki for the Inner Child, Reiki for the Higher Self.

Philosophy   By using the distance-treatment symbol the boundaries of time and space which rule in the material world can be transcended. The effects of Reiki can be applied at practically any distance without diminishing their power.

What Works? What Doesn't?

If a person is more available to Reiki when actually touched, the distant healing treatment, even over a number of sessions, will be less effective than contact treatment. However this is unusual. Distant healing treatment is generally the remedy of choice for people with strong fears of closeness or being touched.

Experiences My first experience with Reiki distant healing treatment caused me to register for the 2nd Degree in which this technique is also imparted. A young woman was suffering with abdominal inflammation (peritonitis). She could hardly walk due to the pain. After a blood sedimentation her physician recommended hospitalization and an urgent operation. That evening I treated her by laying on my hands while our Reiki Master performed a 30-minute distant healing treatment at the same time. During the entire treatment I could feel an enormous force at work. When the session was over the young woman fell asleep. The following morning all of the symptoms had disappeared and a new examination by the physician gave her a clean bill of health.

Distant Healing Treatment with Reiki

Prerequisite:
2nd Reiki Degree

Technical Instructions

The distant healing treatment with the help of Reiki symbols of the 2nd Degree has many different variations. Below is a list of some of the methods that I have tried out personally with a lot of success. There are certainly many others techniques for distant healing treatment that work just as well. Buddha's guiding principle also applies here: "Truth is what works!"

Distant healing treatment, 1st Method:

Step 1: Draw the distance-treatment symbol and mentally say the corresponding Mantra three times.

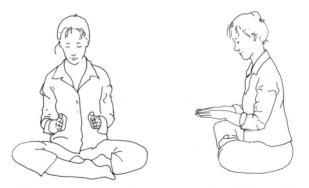

The distance-treatment symbol is the bridge through time and space ...

Step 2: Repeat the names of the person to be treated three times.

Step 3: Visualize the person to be treated. The clearer the image the better.

Step 4: Draw the mental-healing symbol and repeat the Mantra three times.

Step 5: Stabilize everything with the power symbol (draw it once and say the Mantra three times).

Step 6: Fold your hands in front of your heart (palms facing each other) and imagine a miniature of your client to be between them.

Step 7: Begin the treatment. Let yourself be guided by your hands or follow a systematic whole-body treatment.

The treatment should not last longer than 15 minutes if you have difficulty in concentrating.

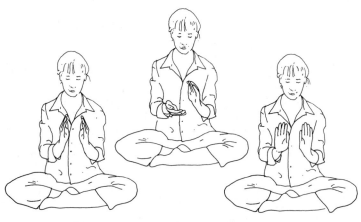

It connects you with your client in the present

Step 8: After the treatment thank your client and rub your hands very intensely for one minute in order to separate from him.

Step 9: Wash your hands.

Additional Technique: If you have learned the Japanese Reiki techniques of Dr. Mikao Usui cleanse yourself with the Kenyoku technique.

Distant healing treatment, 2nd Method:

Step 1: Draw the distance-treatment symbol once and mentally repeat the corresponding Mantra three times.

Step 2: Repeat the name of your client three times.

Step 3: Draw the mental-healing symbol and repeat the Mantra three times.

Step 4: Stabilize everything with the power symbol (draw it once and say the Mantra three times).

Step 5: Give yourself a treatment and imagine while you do so that you are treating your client.

Step 6: Let yourself be guided by your hands or follow a systematic whole-body treatment.
The treatment should not be longer than 15 minutes if you have difficulty in concentrating

Step 7: After the treatment thank your client and rub your hands together very intensely for a minute in order to separate from him.

Step 8: Wash your hands.

Additional Technique: If you have learned the Japanese Reiki techniques of Dr. Mikao Usui cleanse yourself with the Kenyoku technique.

Dr. Mikao Usui's Distant Healing Treatment

Step 1: Hold a photo of the person to be treated in your hand or place it in front of you.

Step 2: On the reverse side write their full name and birth date as well as any other helpful information if you don't know them.

Step 3: Draw the distance-treatment symbol once and mentally repeat the corresponding Mantra three times.

Step 4: Repeat the name of your client three times.

Step 5: Let yourself be guided by your hands. The treatment should not be longer than 15 minutes if you have difficulty concentrating.

Step 6: After the treatment thank your client.

Step 7: Cleanse yourself with the Kenyoku technique.

In case you don't have a photo available:

Step 1: Draw a stick-man to represent the client on your knee or on your finger.

Step 2: Draw the distance-treatment symbol once and repeat the corresponding Mantra three times mentally.

Step 3: Repeat the name of your client three times.

Step 4: Let your hands be guided as you treat the stick figure.
The length of the treatment should not exceed 15 minutes.

Step 5: Thank your client.

Step 6: Cleanse yourself with the Kenyoku technique.

Hawayo Takata's Distant Healing Treatment :

Step 1: Invoke the person or situation that needs to be healed three times. Hold your hands parallel to each other at eye level and say: "Present yourself now between my hands."

Step 2: Say: "I bless the Divine within you. This healing energy is given in love. It is up to you to accept or reject it."

Step 3: Draw the power symbol, the distance-treatment symbol and the power symbol once again on the face of the person or situation repeating the appropriate Mantras.

Step 4: Now place this on a previously selected object such as a teddy bear, doll or pillow. This object will now represent the person to be treated. Imagine the head of the client on the left side if you are right-handed. If you are left-handed then do it exactly the other way around.

Step 5: Point to the representative object and say: "I hereby transfer your form to this object."

Step 6: Draw the power symbol on the entire body of the representative and leave a hand on its head as you do so.

Step 7: Begin the treatment at the solar plexus. From here work toward the Dantien and then move toward the heart. If thoughts, feelings or images should arise during the work make a note of them. In your mind ask the client whether there are any other places that still should be treated. If the response is "yes" draw the power symbol above the additional places to be treated.

Step 8: Turn the representative over and treat the head positions.

Step 9: Draw the power symbol (with Mantras) above the crown chakra and continue with the hand positions for the head.

Inserted Additional Technique (Use when Necessary):

To speak with the subconscious mind of the client to better understand him and his difficulties draw the mental-healing symbol and the power symbol above his crown chakra. Along with the Mantras say three times: "May I please speak with the subconscious mind of the client? Does the subconscious mind have something to tell the conscious mind?" Now be alert and open for information. Put complete trust in your intuition here and have pen and paper ready to write down the information. Thank the subconscious mind for its help.

I personally would go through whatever information arises once more very precisely and only reveal to the client what I consider to be relevant and helpful.

This way of working can be used to open the client to past lives. To do this draw the power symbol and the distance-treatment symbol above the crown chakra as described above.

This technique is very powerful and should be used with care. When you work with the 'Emperor's invisible clothes', you must be sure that you are well grounded and that your client can accept and digest what might come to light through such a session.

The best technique is useless if it doesn't have a lasting effect. Fireworks may be interesting to watch but in the end they are just sound and smoke.

After Ending the Additional Technique:

Step 10: Turn the representative object over, the head facing either to the left or to the right and draw the power symbol along the entire length of the body. If you are treating the legs turn the representative to a position that is easy for you to work with. Draw the power symbol above the legs and continue the treatment.

Step 11: Turn the representative around again and express your thanks.

Step 12: Bless your client and take leave of him.

Distant Healing Treatment on the Telephone:

This is a technique that I particularly like. To do this one you use the telephone connection as a bridge to your client. Tell the person you are on the phone with to get comfortable as the treatment will last for about ten minutes and not to hang up during this time. If you want to clarify something during the process speak softly. Here is the technique:

Step 1: Draw the distance-treatment symbol once and mentally repeat the Mantra three times.

Step 2: Repeat the name of your client three times.

Step 3: Draw the mental-healing symbol once and repeat the Mantra three times.

Step 4: Stabilize everything with the power symbol, draw it once and say the Mantra three times.

Step 5: Allow your hands to guide you or follow a systematic whole-body treatment.
If you have difficulty concentrating the length of the treatment should not exceed 15 minutes.

Step 6: After the treatment thank your client and rub your hands together vigorously for a minute in order to separate.

Step 7: Wash your hands.

Additional Technique: If you have learned the Japanese Reiki techniques of Dr. Mikao Usui cleanse yourself with the Kenyoku technique (from *The Original Reiki Handbook of Dr. Mikao Usui,* Lotus Press.)

Length	10 to 15 minutes.
Please Note	It is necessary to rest afterwards. The client should not drive in traffic or do risky work calling for full attention during or shortly after the distant healing treatment. A follow-up conversation on the phone is a good practice. If you did not take notes during the treatment speak with your client within the next 20 minutes or so before you forget what you noticed. Subsequent communication between sender and recipient is very important especially for beginners since both gain in confidence through the exchange as they notice that distant healing treatment actually works!
Use	With this technique you can send energy through time and space. This means that you can also provide other people, animals, plants and places with energy.
	In this way you can treat parts of the body (your own for example) that you cannot reach or do not want to touch.
Combination	When an on-site treatment is not always possible you can combine the distant healing treatment and the whole-body treatment.
Philosophy	The distant healing treatment may seem quite far-fetched at first glance but lots happens at a distance these days. We live in an age where we are surrounded by an ocean of waves: radio waves, television waves, microwaves, cell-phone waves and computer waves just to mention a few. Even the hairdryer, the electric shaver, and the desk lamp flood us with their electromagnetic waves.

A hundred years ago every modern electrician would have been thrown into the loony bin. Just the claim that pictures would be running wildly on a glass monitor in every living room would have been enough to have you committed.

Our thoughts are also waves. They easily transcend time and space. We have all had this type of experience: You dream an unknown face and three days later you meet this very person. You think of someone you know and there they are suddenly standing at your front door or next to you at the supermarket checkout.

In all cultures of the world people know that thoughts can be sent. In our dim, dark past evil thoughts were often transmitted in this way. But what works with evil thoughts also works with beneficial ones!

When something formless is packaged in a form it works even better. We are familiar with this approach from voodoo dolls but think also of the Buddha statue or the image of Christ. The energy is given a form so that we can feel it and use it. The same thing happens in a Reiki distant healing treatment.

What Works? What Doesn't?

As described above we can work beyond the limits of time and space with the help of this technique. It is a big help but it can also be misused.

The most important rule on the topic of distant healing treatment is this: Only treat a person who has expressly asked for it. The line between help and manipulation is very fine.

I am often asked through the Internet to send someone Reiki. My first question is always: "Does the person really want this?" In 95 cases out of 100 I never hear a word again. We can save ourselves a lot of time like this!

A wonderful way to be free of the constant need to ask permission is to make a 'Reiki agreement' with a group of friends that allows each one to send Reiki to the others at any time.

Experiences

My experiences with this technique could fill an entire book. One story spontaneously comes to mind as I write and I would like to share it with you.

The eight-year-old son of friends in New York had been tormented for years by occasional but vehement bouts of asthma. Over a period of several weeks I treated him with distance Reiki. The asthma disappeared and has not returned to this day, five years later. And it will not return ....

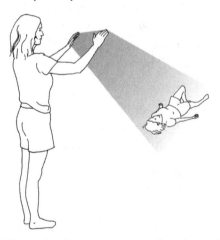

During a Reiki distant healing treatment the client lies or sits in a relaxed position so that optimal opening to Reiki energy can happen

Electrical Appliances—Charging with Reiki

Prerequisite:

2nd Reiki Degree

Technical Instructions

Step 1: Sit down comfortably and take a few deep breaths.

Step 2: Draw the distance-treatment symbol once and mentally repeat the corresponding Mantra three times.

Step 3: Now say the name or description of the appliance to be treated three times plus: "I hereby store the Reiki energy in ... (name of the ob-

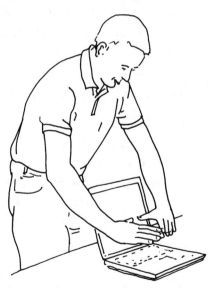

This will definitely be a good book

149

ject). Every time that this device is turned on the Reiki energy will flow." While you say this concentrate on your third eye.

Step 4: Now draw the mental-healing symbol once and repeat the Mantra three times.

Step 5: Seal everything with the power symbol (draw it once and repeat the Mantra three times).

Length   2 to 5 minutes.

Please Note   If you would like to treat electrical appliances directly please do this either with the object unplugged or by touching parts that do not have current running through them.

Use   This technique is used to store Reiki in articles of daily use. When the device is turned on the Reiki energy is also reactivated.
For example, in hot countries Reiki can be stored in ventilators or air-conditioning systems. Radios, cars and juicers can also be treated in this manner.

Combination   Distant healing treatment, Objects—Treating with Reiki.

Philosophy   Energy flows through the entire universe. Thoughts are energy and as human beings we potentially have the power to manifest specific thoughts. Dr. Mikao Usui called human beings "the most highly developed beings in existence."

What Works? What Doesn't?

This technique can easily be 'misused.' Always ask yourself why you want to program an object in the future. In most cases it is advisable to decide which path you want to take in the moment. The future is not predictable. Everything flows and changes according to rules with which we are not familiar and which do not follow us, but rather a higher principle. Thank God!

Experiences   Friends of mine in Malaysia store Reiki in their ventilators. Every time that the ventilator is turned on they say the energy begins to flow. I have not personally tried out this variation.

Emotional Problems—Treating with Reiki

Prerequisite:
2nd Reiki Degree

Technical Instructions

Step 1: Draw the mental-healing symbol once above the client's heart chakra and silently repeat the corresponding Mantra three times.

Step 2: Seal everything with the power symbol. As you do this draw the symbol in the usual way once and silently repeat the Mantra three times. Physically push the symbol into the heart chakra and let it flow out of the palms of your hands for 30 seconds.

Step 3: Now give Reiki to the heart chakra for 5 to 10 minutes.

Length   5 to 10 minutes.

Please Note   This technique acts effectively to control emotional pain. If you should need to use it every day then you know that other measures are also necessary.

Use   This technique works wonders in times of emotional crises or moodiness.

Combination   Whole-body treatment, mental healing, deprogramming.

Philosophy   Emotional crises are not our natural state of being. There can be no fundamental objection to sadness and pain, and the simplest method of defusing them is simply to accept them as they are. If you have to cry then do so! Naturally there are situations where it may not be appropriate and this technique is helpful. By using it we turn to our own essence. The moment we do this the world is seen as fine just as it is.

What Works? What Doesn't?

With this technique we can help our clients return to their natural state of being. The effect does however diminish over time. If the crisis is based on a more deep-rooted problem which manifests over and over again then together with our client we need to try to find its cause. Symptoms are indications that the body or the psyche send us. Be thankful for them!

Experiences   For many years now I have systematically used this technique whenever I simply don't feel good. The effect often appears within a matter of seconds.

Food and Drinks—Charging with Reiki 1

Prerequisite:

1st Reiki Degree

Technical Instructions

Step 1: Sit down comfortably and take a few deep breaths.

Step 2: Take the food in question in your hands or hold your hands 2 to 4 inches above it.

Step 3: Let the energy flow for one to three minutes, or until you feel that it is enough.

Length 2 to 5 minutes.

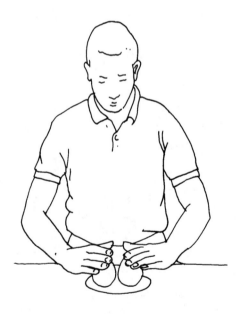

Please Note   Reiki is not a miracle fix that makes spoiled food edible again!

Use   This technique is used to energize food that is lacking in energy or has been prepared without love. Experiment with it during the next unavoidable visit to a fast-food restaurant. I don't use it at home or at friends' homes since I think it is presumptuous to question a meal that has been cooked with love.

Combination   Distant healing treatment, working with Reiki, such as cooking with Reiki.

Philosophy   Foods, especially those that are fresh and organically cultivated, react very joyfully to Reiki. But you can treat all types of foods, nutritional supplements, vitamins, drinks etc with this technique.

What Works? What Doesn't?

Food that is unhealthy or no longer fit to eat cannot be made healthy and edible with Reiki. I know someone who sits in the lotus position when he drinks sake so that his left foot energizes his liver! That's like slapping yourself in the face with one hand and stroking yourself with the other.

Yet we can have a very positive influence on the energy of foods with Reiki.

Experiences   A friend of mine who is a Reiki teacher runs an Italian restaurant in Sapporo. When I am off color (and naturally even when I am in great physical shape) I let myself be healed by him and his art of cooking. It always works!

155

Food and Drinks—Charging with Reiki 2

Prerequisite:

2nd Reiki Degree

Technical Instructions

Step 1: Sit down comfortably and take a few deep breaths.

Step 2: Draw the distance-treatment symbol once and mentally repeat the *corresponding Mantra three times.*

Step 3: Now repeat the name and the location of the food to be treated three times.

Step 4: In your mind draw the mental-healing symbol once above the food or envelop it in a mental-healing-symbol pyramid (to do this draw the mental-healing symbol above the food and create an energy pyramid over it with both hands). Repeat the Mantra for both variations three times.

Step 5: Now seal everything with the power symbol, draw it once and repeat the Mantra three times.

Step 6: Let the energy flow ....

Length   2 to 5 minutes, longer if necessary.

Please Note   Spoiled food belongs on the compost pile!

Use   This technique is used to treat food by means of distance Reiki.

156

Combination Distant healing treatment, Food and Drinks—
Charging with Reiki 1.

Philosophy Any food is open to Reiki distant healing treatment in the same way as human beings and an-
imals. It gratefully absorbs the energy sent which
then benefits the person who eats this nourishment. Human beings, animals and the plant
world are all connected with each other.

What Works? What Doesn't?

This technique is intended to enrich with energy and love food that is located in other places.
I don't know whether it is possible to prolong
the expiration date of food in this way and I don't
have any special desire to experiment!

Experiences A year ago Walter and I visited a holy man in
northern India. As he offered us the *prasad,* consecrated sweets in keeping with the Indian cus-
tom, I smelled something strange. The sweets
were just as sweet but also just as old as the holy
man sitting before us clad only in a canvas sack.
Although I used this technique I was also happy
to accept a small homeopathic remedy from
Walter afterwards. Fortunately neither of us got
sick from this little adventure.

Future Situations—Treating with Reiki

Prerequisite:

2nd Reiki Degree

Technical Instructions

I like to compare this technique to the way we program a video recorder so as to record a specific future program in our absence.

Step 1: Sit comfortably and take a few deep breaths.

Step 2: Draw the distance-treatment symbol once and mentally repeat the corresponding Mantra three times.

Step 3: Repeat the name or the description of the situation that you want to provide with Reiki three times. Say: "Please give energy to this situation from ... (the beginning time) to ... (the ending time)."

Step 4: Draw the mental-healing symbol once, repeat the Mantra three times and send it to the situation.

Step 5: Seal everything with the power symbol (draw it once and repeat the Mantra three times).

Length 10 to 15 minutes.

Please Note If you are treating another person you should, of course have the recipient's permission to send them Reiki. If you send Reiki to a situation in the future in which you and other people are involved send the energy to yourself only.

In another way, just like lighting a candle in a church you can use Reiki as an offering. In this case send Reiki to the situation and say: "May this energy be received by those who would like to absorb it."

Use It is used for enriching future situations with Reiki.

Combination Distant healing treatment whole-body treatment affirmation technique (deprogramming with Reiki).

Philosophy Past present and future are three parts of a perpetual harmonious whole.
P. D. Ouspensky a student of the Russian mystic Georg I. Gurdjieff explains the phenomenon of time in one of his books like this: Time is like a wheel filled with many spokes. In our normal state of consciousness we perceive one of the spokes at a any given moment even though all of the other spokes are also present *at the same time.* This means that past, present and future are one. Thus we can successfully work with Reiki on all three levels of time.

What Works? What Doesn't?

Reiki supports the highest good for everyone involved in a situation. Sometimes we don't get the job that we wanted because we can learn more somewhere else. For the same reason sometimes our suffering is not relieved.

But we can be sure that in the greater plan of things the best is intended for us. In the words of the Indian sage Sri Ramakrishna: "Give God (or existence) the power over all the decisions in your life. Then you will be truly happy."

Experiences In my experience this technique works wonderfully when you sit totally relaxed in the bathtub and treat a situation in the future as you do so.

Grounding with the Power Symbol

Prerequisite:

2nd Reiki Degree

Technical Instructions

Step 1: Stand in a relaxed fashion with both feet parallel to each other and take several deep breaths.

Step 2: Now draw the power symbol once and send it into both of your hand chakras in the center of the palms. Repeat the corresponding Mantra three times mentally.

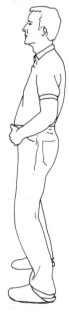

Life is better when you are grounded

When I do this I imagine stamping the symbol into the palms of my hands. This may be easier to do with each hand separately. After you have done it several times you can send the symbol into both hand chakras at the same time.

Step 3: Draw the power symbol once again and send it into one of your foot chakras in the center of the sole of the foot. Repeat the Mantra three times.

Step 4: Now send the symbol into the other foot and repeat the Mantra three times.
After you have done this several times you can send the symbol into both feet at the same time.

Step 5: Now draw the power symbol once again in your mind and send it into your Dantien. Silently repeat the Mantra three times.

Variation: Draw the power symbol once in each of your hand chakras, your foot chakras and your *Dantien*. Each time you do this repeat the Mantra of the symbols silently three times.

Length	1 to 2 minutes.
Please Note	For chronic grounding problems I recommend hard physical labor as well as regular Reiki treatments in the region of the belly, the knees and the ankles.
Use	This technique can help ground you and keep you there. Whenever you do not feel centered or if your knees get shaky before an unpleasant meeting like a job interview or some type of con-

frontation you can use this technique. You can dance into any situation in life in a relaxed and grounded way and be at your very best with this technique.

Combination   This technique can be combined with the treatment of the ankles, the knees and the *Dantien*.

Philosophy   Whenever we are not rooted with both legs firmly in the earth we cannot stretch our crown to the sky. A farmer certainly does not need this type of grounding but Reiki teachers in particular who deal in ethereal matters must be sure that the other end of the spectrum also gets its due. Only a *whole* human being can be balanced and happy.

What Works? What Doesn't?

With this technique we can put ourselves in the best shape imaginable to deal with life's situations. It really doesn't help wanting to avoid potential difficulties. They exist so that we can look them squarely in the eye and grow from the experience.

Experiences   After practicing this technique for many years it has become such a part of me that I no longer have to make any effort to ground myself.

Healing Stones—Activating with Rainbow Reiki

Prerequisite:

1st Reiki Degree

Technical Instructions

> *Step 1:* Take the healing stones to be activated between your hands and hold them for a moment. Feel their specific vibrations and make contact with them.

> *Step 2:* Open your hands upward with the stones facing the sky and look up also.

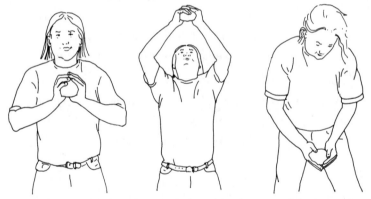

Activating a healing stone with the spiritual powers of the heart, heaven and earth

> *Step 3:* Sing the Mantra "Hey Loa, Key Loa, Manaho, Lo" at least nine times.

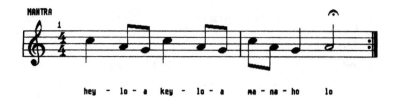

hey - lo - a key - lo - a na - na - ho lo

Step 4: Holding the stones turn your hands down towards the earth and also look in this direction.

Step 5: Sing the Mantra "Hey Loa, Key Loa, Manaho, Lo" at least nine times.

Step 6: Hold your hands in front of your heart.

Step 7: Sing the Mantra "Hey Loa, Key Loa, Manaho, Lo" at least nine times.

Step 8: Thank Father Sky and Mother Earth or, put another way, God and the Goddess for allowing their children, the healing stones, to come to you.

Step 9: Ask them to bless the healing stones and to bless you so that you can treat and use them in a spiritual way.

Length

In my experience depending on the tempo with which you sing it this exercise lasts about 5 to 8 minutes.

Please Note

The Mantra can easily be repeated more than nine times, but not less since the effect of this technique will otherwise be greatly diminished.

Use

For the activation of healing stones. Stones that are especially well suited are quartz crystals, fluorite, amethyst, rose quartz, moss agate, citrine, smoky quartz, rhodochrosite, thulite and carnelian.

Combination   Crystal healing with Rainbow Reiki, crystal fountains with Rainbow Reiki, Rainbow Reiki crystal mandalas*.

Philosophy   The Rainbow Reiki healing Mantra comes from the ancient spiritual tradition of the continent of Lemuria which sank in the Pacific Ocean after being hit by a gigantic meteorite. The Mantra calls upon the presence of the creative force and its kind angels, inviting them to participate in whatever is unfolding at the moment.

This deeply effective spiritual influence activates objects like healing stones in a way similar to the activation of the source substances of the homeopathic remedies of Samuel Hahnemann. In this way much more comprehensive healing powers are released than would normally be possible in the inactivated state. Many of the effects attributed to healing stones can only be observed when they have been activated.

In this technique Reiki fulfills the task of increasing the frequency of the stones quickly and opens them more intensively for activation. This works especially well with healing stones that have been placed under a strong Reiki shower overnight.

What Works? What Doesn't?

Any stone, mineral or crystal, a pebble found in the forest or a diamond of jewelry quality can

---

* Some of the most effective Rainbow Reiki crystal mandalas are to be found in my book *Rainbow Reiki*, published by Lotus Press.

have its healing power increased and refined to a high degree through the Rainbow Reiki healing-stone activation. Yet this does not negate the importance of other techniques, patience in the practice or good contact between the healer and the client.

Experiences Pets almost always go to drink from a water bowl with an activated quartz crystal rather than one with a non-activated crystal. Be sure to orient the point correctly.

Homeopathic Touch with Reiki

Prerequisite:

1st Reiki Degree

Technical Instructions

Step 1: Gently touch the area to be treated.

Step 2: Make circling and stroking movements in different directions, keeping them very gentle, calm and slow. While doing this let yourself be guided more by your intuition and capacity for understanding than by your mind.

Step 3: In closing, move your hands gently away from the surface of the body.

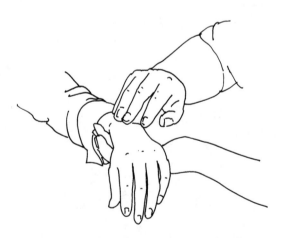

Opening the body for Reiki with gentle touch

Length	Between 30 seconds and 5 minutes, depending on how strongly the area to be treated is blocked and the intensity of the Reiki treatment desired.
Please Note	The movements really must be very gentle, calm and even. Treat injured areas only in the aura at a distance of about one handwidth.
Use	Increasing the receptivity for Reiki. Improved exchange of energy between the treated area and with the rest of the body.
Combination	Whole-body treatment, special positions, systematic chakra work, intuitive Reiki, distant healing treatment, crystal treatment with Reiki.
Philosophy	According to the Arndt-Schulze Law* of psychiatry and biocybernetics a small amount of stimulation promotes life activity while large quantities inhibit it. Great amounts paralyze or have a destructive influence. With the gentle, calm stimulus of the homeopathic touch we kindle life activity. The attention of the body's consciousness is directed to the area treated in this way. Life energy flows wherever attention is directed. This way the area treated by the homeopathic touch is reintegrated into the energetic metabolism of the body. This almost always leads to an increase in circulation and a substantial overall improvement in the incorporation of the areas treated into the body's metabolism.
	The still rather young science of psycho-neuroimmunology has in recent decades collected much

---

* Rudolf Arndt-Schulze, psychiatrist, Greifswald/Germany, 1835-1900.

evidence on the positive effect of the gentle, calm touch on human health.

What Works? What Doesn't?

The receptivity of the body can be tremendously increased with the homeopathic touch. As a result Reiki can achieve more extensive and faster effects. At the same time in most cases it is not possible to use this technique alone to completely eliminate strong fears, deep-rooted dogmas and similar major blocks which may be counteracting healing. Recommended approaches for this purpose are clarifying conversations and the use of other Reiki methods such as KarmaClearing, mental healing and systematic chakra healing.

Experiences Techniques such as the homeopathic touch and the opening of the chakras can be especially decisive in successfully treating chronic health disorders. Stuck emotions and old traumas that have been encapsulated within the musculature often require these techniques in order to be resolved and harmonized.

Karma-Cleansing with Reiki

Prerequisite:

2nd Reiki Degree

Technical Instructions

Step 1: Draw the distance-treatment symbol once and mentally repeat the corresponding Mantra three times.

Step 2: Repeat three times the name of your client, the situation, the place or the term for what you would like to heal.

Step 3: Draw the mental-healing symbol once and repeat the Mantra three times.

Step 4: Stabilize everything with the power symbol (draw it once, say the Mantra three times).

Step 5: Apologize to the other person.

Step 6: Give Reiki to the situation.

Step 7: After the treatment use the Kenyoku technique or rub your hands together briskly for a minute to separate from your client.

Length

10 to 15 minutes for at least one week every day or until you have the feeling that the matter is completed.

Please Note

It is a good idea to rest after the treatment. During or shortly after the session you should not drive in traffic or do risky work that calls for your complete concentration.

After the treatment it may be advisable to talk to someone you trust. This technique can cause unpleasant things from the past to the surface. Be prepared for tears and strong feelings.

Use This technique is the perfect tool to treat a situation from your childhood or from a past life.

Combination Healing the childhood self, work with the Inner Child, the Reiki Box, Reiki Essences, Karma-Clearing with Rainbow Reiki (see page 174), whole-body treatment.

Philosophy We are the product of our entire past experiences. These experiences are very complex as we all know. They seem good and bad, healthy and unhealthy, beautiful and cruel. Whatever they may be they have shaped us and brought us into this moment with all of its peaks and valleys.

While some of these experiences may have left a bitter taste, this technique gives us a method for finding relief.

What Works? What Doesn't?

What has happened can never be undone.

Using this technique we can however integrate unpleasant experiences thereby transforming them for our benefit. Life does not recognize our contrived moral concepts, it acknowledges energy. And this energy is beyond good and evil, beyond judgment.

If you still have something unresolved with someone make an effort to 'clean up' the karma with him or her. If this person is no longer alive or you have lost track of them Karma-Cleansing is the right technique.

Karma-Cleansing does not mean that we can undo something that has happened. When my girlfriend committed suicide 25 years ago my pain and feelings of guilt were so overwhelming that I could not deal with them. Later though I was able to face them with the help of this technique. I spent several weeks in hot tears with great feelings of love, and through this grieving the knot in my heart was unraveled.

KarmaClearing with Rainbow Reiki

Prerequisite:

2nd Reiki Degree

Technical Instructions

A Tip: Although the instructions for this technique may appear quite simple it is quite complex. It will be easier for you to practice the sequence at the appropriate speed if you read the instructions into a tape recorder and then use this recording to direct you. Of course you could also have a friend read the individual steps to you.

Variation 1: Rainbow Reiki KarmaClearing for Yourself

Step 1: Draw the distance-treatment symbol and activate it by saying or thinking its Mantra three times.

Step 2: Draw the power symbol and activate it with the Mantra three times.

Step 3: Then say three times: "Inner Child of ... (your first and last name)."

Step 4: Draw several power symbols for your Inner Child* and activate each of them with the Mantra three times. This will cause more Reiki to flow to your Inner Child and it will help give you better support.

---

* If you are not yet familiar with the Rainbow Reiki technique of 'Rainbow Reiki for the Inner Child,' please read the explanation of it on page 244.

Step 5: Draw the distance-treatment symbol and activate it with the Mantra three times.

Step 6: Draw the power symbol and activate it with its Mantra three times.

Step 7: Then say or think three times: "Higher Self of ... (your first and last name)."

Step 8: Draw several power symbols for your Higher Self* and activate each of them with the Mantra three times. This will cause more Reiki to flow to your Higher Self and help give you better support.

Step 9: Ask your Inner Child and your Higher Self for support in the following KarmaClearing.

Step 10: Draw the distance-treatment symbol and activate it with its Mantra three times.

Step 11: Draw the power symbol and activate it with the Mantra three times.

Step 12: Say your first and last name three times while you visualize your own face.

Step 13: Now imagine yourself as a small-scale body between your hands with the head up, the feet down and the face toward you.

Step 14: Draw several power symbols above your miniature body between your hands and activate each symbol by its Mantra three times.** This will cause more Reiki to flow to you. This supports your receptivity for the pleasant effects of KarmaClearing.

---

* If you are not yet familiar with the Rainbow Reiki technique of 'Rainbow Reiki for the Higher Self' please read the explanation on page 241.

** If you are not yet familiar with the Rainbow Reiki technique of 'Distance Healing' please read the explanation on pages 133-137.

It will also help you integrate or eliminate the released energies and structures and increase your vibration level which will make it easier for you to open up to the astral energy work.

Step 15: Now ask your Inner Child to help you on its subtle level. Take its hand by stretching one of your physical hands upward and grasp its energetic hand through the appropriate movement. Pull yourself up on it and climb to the subtle level with your energy body.

Step 16: Imagine that there is a line beginning at your current position, here and now. This line runs into the past and is symbolic of your life up to the present. It is enough to simply say this in words, but if you can 'see' it in your mind's eye so much the better. Do not limit it. The life process is infinite because its origin is divine. No beginning, no end.

Step 17: Now there are two possibilities. You can work in a general way which is explained here as Procedure A. Given regularly this type of Rainbow Reiki KarmaClearing is very useful as spiritual psycho-hygiene as long as there are no major difficulties that need attention. Procedure B explains how you can apply yourself to a specific topic with the Rainbow Reiki KarmaClearing.

Procedure A: Ask your Inner Child and your Higher Self to show you a trauma (emotional injury) that has not yet healed. Ask for it to be shown as a dark spot, a cross, a circle or some other distinct symbol on your timeline. This should be a trauma whose healing at this point is both meaningful and useful which will also involve as little risk as possible for you in the healing process.

Procedure B: Ask your Inner Child and your Higher Self to show you a trauma (emotional injury) that is the original cause of a specific problem in your life that has not yet healed. Ask for it to be shown to you as a dark spot, a cross, a circle or some other distinct symbol on your timeline. This should be a trauma whose healing at this point is especially meaningful and useful, which will also involve as little risk as possible for you in the healing process.

Step 18: The next procedure is the same in both cases. Immediately after you have spoken your request imagine that there is a corresponding mark on your timeline that symbolizes a trauma.

Step 19: With plenty of distance from your timeline move along it into the past. In no case should you step on your timeline.

Step 20: Stop at the mark that symbolizes the trauma and build a Reiki shower above it by drawing a distance-treatment symbol above the mark. Then activate it by saying its Mantra three times. Draw several power symbols that have one flat side facing the distance-treatment symbol and the other flat side toward the mark of the trauma. Activate the symbol by saying it three times. On no account should you attempt to enter the dark spot or learn more about its contents! This would not intensify the effect of the Rainbow Reiki KarmaClearing. As long as you follow this rule the method is very safe and can do much good.

Step 21: Return to your starting point (current position) and let your Inner Child lead you back to the level of everyday life. Let it help you back into your physical body. To do this give it your hand and allow your energy body to merge with your physical form through an appropriate symbolic movement.

Step 22: Thank your Inner Child and your Higher Self for their support and take leave of them in the usual way. Then take leave of the distance contact with yourself.

Variation 2:
Rainbow Reiki KarmaClearing for Another Person

Step 1: Draw the distance-treatment symbol and activate it by saying or thinking its Mantra three times.

Step 2: Draw the power symbol and activate it with its Mantra three times.

Step 3: Then say or think three times: "Inner Child of ... (your first and last name)."

Step 4: Draw several power symbols for your Inner Child and activate each of them by saying the Mantra three times. This will cause more Reiki to flow to your Inner Child and it will help give you better support.

Step 5: Draw the distance-treatment symbol and activate it with its Mantra three times.

Step 6: Draw the power symbol and activate it with its Mantra three times.

Step 7: Then say or think three times: "Higher Self of ... (your first and last name)."

Step 8: Draw several power symbols for your Higher Self and activate each of them by saying the Mantra three times. This will cause more Reiki to flow to your Higher Self and this will help it to give you better support.

Step 9: Draw the distance-treatment symbol and activate it with its Mantra three times.

Step 10: Draw the power symbol and activate it with its Mantra three times.

Step 11: Now say or think three times: "Inner Child of ... (first and last name of the person to be treated)."

Step 12: Draw several power symbols for the Inner Child and activate each of them with its Mantra three times.

Step 13: Draw the distance-treatment symbol and activate it with its Mantra three times.

Step 14: Draw the power symbol and activate it with its Mantra three times.

Step 15: Now say or think three times: "Higher Self of ... (first and last name of the person to be treated)."

Step 16: Draw several power symbols for the Higher Self and activate each of them with the Mantra three times.

Step 17: Ask your Inner Child and your Higher Self as well as the Inner Child and the Higher Self of the person to be treated for support in the following KarmaClearing.

Step 18: Draw the distance-treatment symbol and activate it with its Mantra three times.

Step 19: Draw the power symbol and activate it with its Mantra three times.

Step 20: Say or think the first and last names the person to be treated three times while you visualize his/her face.

Step 21: Now imagine your client as a miniature body between your hands with the head up, the feet down and the face toward you.

Step 22: Draw several power symbols above the small-scale body between your hands and activate each symbol by saying its Mantra three times.

Step 23: Ask your Inner Child to help you onto the subtle level of your client where you can work with the timeline. Take its hand by stretching your physical hand upward and grasping its energetic hand through a suitable movement. Then pull your-self up and climb into the subtle level with your energy body.

Step 24: Imagine that there is a line beginning at your client's current position, here and now. This line runs into the past and is symbolic of your client's life up to the present. It is enough to simply say this in words, but if you can 'see' it in your mind's eye so much the better. Do not limit it. The life process is infinite because its origin is divine. No beginning, no end.

Step 25: Now there are two possibilities: You can work in a gen-eral way which is explained under Procedure A. If there are no major difficulties in your client's life requiring attention this type of Rainbow Reiki KarmaClearing is good as regular spiritual psycho-hygiene. Procedure B explains how you can harmonize a specific topic with the Rainbow Reiki KarmaClearing.

Procedure A: Ask the Inner Child and Higher Self of your client to show you a trauma (emotional injury) that has not yet healed. Ask for it to show as a dark spot, a cross, a circle or some other distinct symbol on your client's timeline. This should be a trauma whose healing at this point would be especially meaningful and useful, involving little risk for your client.

Procedure B: Ask the Inner Child and Higher Self of your client to show you a trauma (emotional injury) that is the original cause of a specific problem in your client's life that has not yet healed. Ask for it to be indicated as a dark spot, a cross, a circle or some other distinct symbol on your client's timeline. This should be a trauma whose healing at this point would be especially meaningful and useful, and involving little risk for your client.

Step 26: The further procedure is the same in both cases. Immediately after you have spoken your request, imagine that there is a corresponding mark on your client's timeline symbolizing a trauma.

Step 27: With plenty of distance from the timeline move along it into the past. You should never step on the timeline.

Step 28: Stop at the mark that symbolizes the trauma and build a Reiki shower above it by drawing a distance-treatment symbol above it. Then activate it by saying its Mantra three times. Draw several power symbols that have one flat side facing the distance-treatment symbol and the other flat side toward the mark of the trauma. Activate it by saying the Mantra three times.

On no account should you attempt to enter the dark spot or learn more about its contents! This would in not intensify the effect of the Rainbow Reiki KarmaClearing in any way. As long as you follow this rule this method is very safe and can do much good.

Step 29: Return to your starting point (current position—now) and let yourself be led back to the level of everyday life by your Inner Child. Allow it to help you back into your material body. To do this give it your hand and let your energy body merge with your material form through an appropriate symbolic movement.

Step 30: Thank your Inner Child and your Higher Self as well as the client's Inner Child and Higher Self for their support and take leave of them in the usual way. Then take leave of the distance contact with yourself.

Variation 3:
Rainbow Reiki KarmaClearing for a Building

It may seem strange to you that a technique like Rainbow Reiki KarmaClearing also works for an apparently inanimate object like a building. Yet from the spiritual perspective ultimately everything has grown out of the creative force and it actually works. Go ahead and try it out. You may have had the experience that certain buildings feel somehow dead, while others seem rather serious. Others may even feel quite amusing or healing or wise. Everything has its soul. If we respectfully recognize this soul and establish contact with it we can heal it, learn from it and make friends with it.

Step 1: Draw the distance-treatment symbol and activate it by saying or thinking its Mantra three times.

Step 2: Draw the power symbol and activate it by saying its Mantra three times.

Step 3: Then say three times: "Inner Child of ... (your first and last name)."

Step 4: Draw several power symbols for your Inner Child and activate each of them with the Mantra three times. This will cause more Reiki to flow to your Inner Child and it will help it to give you better support.

Step 5: Draw the distance-treatment symbol and activate it with its Mantra three times.

Step 6: Draw the power symbol and activate it with its Mantra three times.

Step 7: Then say or think three times: "Higher Self of ... (your first and last name)."

Step 8: Draw several power symbols for your Higher Self and activate each of them three times. This will cause more Reiki to flow to your Higher Self and this will help it to give you better support.

Step 9: Draw the distance-treatment symbol and activate it by saying or thinking its Mantra three times.

Step 10: Draw the power symbol and activate it with its Mantra three times.

Step 11: Now say or think three times: "Inner Child of ... (name of the building, for example: the name of the town, street and house number)."

Step 12: Draw several power symbols for the Inner Child and activate each of them.

Step 13: Draw the distance-treatment symbol and activate it.

Step 14: Draw the power symbol and activate it.

Step 15: Now say or think three times: "Higher Self of ... (name of the building, for example: the name of the town, the street and house number)."

Step 16: Draw several power symbols for the Higher Self and activate each of them by saying the Mantra three times.

Step 17: Ask your Inner Child and your Higher Self as well as the Inner Child and the Higher Self of the building to be treated for support in the following KarmaClearing.

Step 18: Draw the distance-treatment symbol and activate it with its Mantra three times.

Step 19: Draw the power symbol and activate it.

Step 20: Say or think the name of the building three times while you visualize it.

Step 21: Now imagine the building as a miniature model between your hands with the roof upward and the entrance area facing you.

Step 22: Draw several power symbols above the small-scale building between your hands and activate each symbol three times.

Step 23: Ask your Inner Child to help you access the subtle level of the building where you can work with its timeline. Take its hand by stretching your physical hand upward and grasping its energetic hand through a corresponding movement. Then pull yourself up and rise to the subtle level with your energy body.

Step 24: Imagine that there is a line beginning at this building's current position, here and now. This line runs into the past and is symbolic of the building's life up to the present. It is enough to simply say this in words, but if you can 'see' it in your mind's eye so much the better. Do not limit it. The life process is infinite because its origin is divine. No beginning, no end.

Step 25: Now there are two possibilities: You can work in a general way which is explained here as Procedure A. This type of Rainbow Reiki KarmaClearing is very useful as regular spiritual psycho-hygiene if there are no major problems or difficulties in the life of the building. Procedure B explains how you can harmonize a specific topic with the Rainbow Reiki KarmaClearing.

Procedure A: Ask the Inner Child and Higher Self of your client to show you a trauma (emotional injury) that has not yet healed. Ask for it to show as a dark spot, a cross, a circle or some other distinct symbol on your client's timeline. This should be a trauma whose healing at this point would be especially meaningful and useful, involving little risk for your client.

Procedure B: Ask the Inner Child and Higher Self of the building to show you a trauma (emotional injury) that is the original cause of a specific problem in the building's life that has not yet healed as a dark spot, a cross, a circle or some other distinct symbol on the building's timeline. This should be a trauma whose healing at this time is especially meaningful and useful, involving as little risk as possible for the building.

Step 26: The next procedure is the same in both cases. Immediately after you have spoken your request imagine a corresponding mark on the building's timeline that symbolizes a trauma.

Step 27: With plenty of distance from the timeline move along it into the past. You should never step on the timeline.

Step 28: Stop at the mark that symbolizes the trauma and build a Reiki shower above it by drawing a distance-treatment symbol over it and activating this by saying its Mantra three times. Then draw several power symbols that have one flat side facing the distance-treatment symbol and the other flat side toward the mark of the trauma. Activate its Mantra by saying it three times. In no case should you attempt to enter the dark spot or learn more about its contents! This would not intensify the effect of the Rainbow Reiki KarmaClearing at all. As long as you follow this rule the method is very safe and can do a lot of good.

Step 29: Return to your starting point (current position) and let your Inner Child lead you back to the level of everyday life. Allow it to help you back into your material body. To do this give it your hand and let your energy body merge with your material form through the corresponding movement.

Step 30: Thank your Inner Child and your Higher Self as well as the Inner Child and Higher Self of the building for their support and take leave of them in the usual way. Then take leave of the distance contact with yourself.

Length	Depending on the extent of the KarmaClearing, 15 minutes to an hour or more will be required per session. However 15 to 20 minutes are usually adequate.
Please Note	It is necessary to rest afterwards. During and shortly after the session no work that requires full concentration should be undertaken. It is best for the recipient to be lying down during the session and feel what is going on inside.
Use	Processing trauma from this life and from earlier incarnations, release of blocked abilities and dissolution of stubborn sabotage programs, harmonization of fears, neurotic disorders and other mental-emotional imbalances, as the accompanying treatment for difficult illnesses and injuries.

When applying this to buildings, landscapes and power spots, over time the natural flows of energy can be restored. Possessions and other negative energetic structures can be harmonized. This makes Rainbow Reiki KarmaClearing especially suitable for all types of Feng Shui applications.

In the area of family therapy (family Karma-Clearing) whole new possibilities open up because it can be used to deal with problems spanning a number of generations.

On the basis of the three different examples explained above it will be easy for you to adapt the process appropriately when you work with partners, a family or a power place.

Combination Mental healing, light-body work with Rainbow Reiki, contact with angels, power animals and other divine beings, Reiki healing for the Inner Child, Reiki healing for the Higher Self, Reiki healing for situations of the past.

Philosophy In a very general way the word 'karma' describes the principle of the effect of actions in the material world. Inhabitants of the material level create new structures and expand or destroy the existing ones through their actions. This is an inevitable consequence of the divine law applying to the material plane. Moreover, it can also be very helpful in as much as other people may learn from what one individual has achieved. So each individual can contribute more useful life structures.

However, problems arise when disharmonious patterns are created or when useful ones are destroyed. Each of us is spiritually connected with our actions and their outcomes. This responsibility cannot be taken away from us whether we are conscious of it or not. The more disharmony we create, the more harmony we disturb or destroy, the more resulting disharmony we experience. Frequently there is a certain time lapse.

In this case someone with a little awareness and spiritual understanding will begin to work on creating a balance. He will attempt to create positive karma through constructive actions vis a vis the original disharmony.

There are a great many different, more or less effective ways to achieve this. Under certain conditions a spiritual teacher can also help the student to master specific karmic burdens more quickly.

A completely different way of dealing with karma is to be 'in the world but not of the world'. In some Eastern spiritual traditions this is also called Wu-Wei, action through inaction. When we learn to be both sincere and committed to life, *and* see it as one great divine play we no longer accumulate karma. We do our everyday duties diligently at the same time aware that all aspects are simply components of this great divine game. Contrary to the former state of unconsciousness, we may now learn in a way both effective and supporting of our growth processes. Having come to an understanding of one's divinity as well as one's humanness new laws come into effect.

Dear reader please excuse me if I try to explain the complex issue of karma in so few words and such simplified terms. For the successful practice of Rainbow Reiki KarmaClearing this explanation is completely adequate.

Used regularly and over a longer period of time Rainbow Reiki KarmaClearing promotes both the harmonizing and balancing of disharmonious karma, as well as the process of becoming more conscious.

Here is a brief 'technical explanation' of the effective principles in Rainbow Reiki KarmaClearing: Through the Reiki shower Reiki flows to the encapsulated trauma very intensely for a long period of time, healing it gently, slowly and lastingly.

Combined with committed, constructive decisions and uncompromising actions Rainbow Reiki KarmaClearing can help eliminate major difficulties. Armchair energy work is usually not very helpful. The principle of this practice is: *Ora et labora!** Our commitment in the energy work should be as though everything depends on it. On the material plane too we need to apply ourselves as though everything depends on the work we do with our hands.

Experiences I have seen particular success in KarmaClearing when it involved healing difficult childhood or accident traumas. Difficult chronic illnesses which are often based in traumatic situations not directly accessible to the conscious mind have also been resolved using this technique.

---

* Pray and work!

Light-Body Work with Rainbow Reiki

Prerequisite:

2nd Reiki Degree

Technical Instructions

Variation 1

Step 1: Draw the distance-treatment symbol with your initiated hand and say or think the corresponding Mantra three times.

Step 2: Draw the power symbol and say or think the Mantra three times.

Step 3: Visualize the recipient and say or think three times: "Light body of ... (name of the recipient)."

Step 4: Imagine that you are looking into the recipient with your mental eye until you perceive a radiant point of light.

Step 5: Draw several intensification symbols on this soul-light and activate each symbol by saying its Mantra three times.

Step 6: End the application by taking leave of the recipient, wishing him the blessing of the creative force. Blow vigorously between the palms of your hands (about 4 inches apart) and then rub the palms together.

Variation 2

Step 1: Draw the distance-treatment symbol with the initiated hand and say or think the corresponding Mantra three times.

Step 2: Draw the power symbol and say the Mantra three times.

Step 3: Visualize the recipient and say: "Light body of ... (name of the recipient)."

Step 4: Imagine that you are looking into the recipient with your mental eye until you perceive a radiant point of light.

Step 5: Draw the mental-healing symbol on this soul-light and activate with the Mantra three times.

Step 6: Draw the power symbol on the soul-light and activate it with the Mantra three times.

Step 7: Say or think: "Light is truth, shadow is illusion, awaken the light, healing comes in profusion."*

Step 8: Repeat this affirmation nine times or, when a very strong effect is desired 108 times. After each repetition draw the power symbol on the soul-light and activate it with its Mantra three times.

---

* This affirmation comes from a European family spiritual tradition in which I have been trained. The words are part of a holy and healing message from Mother Earth to Her children. The affirmation is used here in connection with deeply effective healing rituals. It has also proved its worth for many years in Rainbow Reiki.

Step 9: In any case no matter how often you use the affirmation let Reiki flow for at least 10 minutes and use several intensification symbols in order to increase the flow of energy. Draw several power symbols on the soul-light and activate each symbol by saying its Mantra three times.

Step 10: End the application by taking leave of the recipient, wishing him the blessing of the creative force, vigorously blowing between the palms of your hands (about 4 inches apart), and then rubbing the palms together.

Length   At least 10 to 15 minutes.

Please Note   It is helpful to rest afterwards. During or shortly after the session the client should not drive in traffic or do risky work that requires complete concentration. Connecting at the end of each session about experiences that might have occurred during the exercise is meaningful in helping to integrate those experiences, promote a conscious understanding of the transformational experience and calm any fears that may have arisen. Sometimes in closing grounding techniques can be helpful to improve the discharge of released energies.

Use   Mystic experiences, awakening the light body, charging and increasing the vibration of the light body, awakening and expanding the light consciousness, increasing the resonance in relation to the life source, harmonization of deep-rooted karmic burdens, support of the meditation practice, development of extrasensory perception such as clairvoyance, increase of vibrations within the material body as an accompanying treatment for serious illnesses or injuries, mental preparation for comprehensive personal and global transformation processes, for the preparation of rituals and intensive periods of cleansing, to prevent the loss of perspective and spiritual insight in difficult situations and phases of life, as the accompanying treatment for problems of possession and black magic, as protection in times when someone must deal with very difficult environmental conditions, situations, and people, to make learning easier—not only in the spiritual sense, to have a clear mind and spiritual understanding before making important decisions, as preparation for initiation into the 3rd Reiki Degree, for intensifying and harmonizing the learning experiences on the Master path.

Combination   Distant healing treatment, distant healing treatment with a group, Rainbow Reiki KarmaClearing, systematic chakra work, mental healing, healing sessions for the Inner Child, healing sessions for the Higher Self.

Philosophy   The light body of a human being is a special, largely independent part of the energy system that guides and organizes currents of non-polar energies. The non-polar energies include Usui Reiki for example.

The human being is connected to the dimension of divine existence through the light body. This is the seat of the god-human identity. Mantras like *Tat Tvam Asi* activate this area and connect it more strongly with the other levels of existence for human beings and improve its resonance with the creative force, the source of all life. The work with Mantras on the light body is not simple. It requires much patience, intense effort and in the absence of a competent teacher is often dangerous because of the enormous forces that are moved and activated.

The Rainbow Reiki energy work however has a different effect because the ego and other materially limiting human structures are largely bypassed.

What Works? What Doesn't?

The light-body work with Rainbow Reiki can be a 'turbocharger' for spiritual development. However, like all of the other techniques it does not replace contact with a spiritual teacher or personal decisions and their consistent translation into action. Personal responsibility is not bypassed, nor is solid work in the material realm, in relationships or in professional life. It also cannot replace medical training or any other type of training required to deal with special challenges. However Rainbow Reiki light-body work is a unique lever with which all these activities can become more effective. It is very helpful in successfully overcoming difficulties that are too great for conventional methods.

Experiences   I recommend the Rainbow Reiki light-body work to Reiki friends who are keen to give their life a basic spiritual direction and structure. It has also proved helpful in serious life crises.

A friend once told me of a special experience she had in an ancient temple in Thailand while doing this exercise in front of a large Buddha statue. Very soon she felt herself being pulled more and more toward the Buddha until she ultimately dissolved into Him. Then in an altered state of consciousness she had an impressive light experience where she saw her life as an infinite, swirling energy current within a gigantic network of other light-energy currents. This experience changed her whole attitude toward life permanently. She began training as a healer as soon as she returned from her trip. She wants nothing more than to bring to the Earth the light she saw in Thailand.

Lost Objects—Finding

Prerequisite:

2nd Reiki Degree

Technical Instructions

Step 1: Sit down comfortably and take a few deep breaths.

Step 2: Write the name or description of the lost object on a piece of paper.

Step 3: Draw the distance-treatment symbol once on the paper and mentally repeat the corresponding Mantra three times.

Step 4: Repeat the name or description of the object three times and then say: "With the help of the Reiki symbol I ask you to lead me to you."

Step 5: Now draw the mental-healing symbol once and repeat the Mantra three.

Step 6: Seal everything with the power symbol.

Step 7: Put the piece of paper in your pocket and return to your everyday life.

In the course of the day you should be able to remember where the lost object is.

Length   2 to 3 minutes.

Please Note   Often we have to first let go of the lost object inwardly before it can find its way back to us. Find your own Buddha nature!

Use	This technique is used to find anything lost. It is helpful not only in finding objects but also pets that have run away or people who have disappeared.
Combination	Distant healing treatment affirmation technique.
Philosophy	Thoughts constantly repeated take on a life of their own. This is the secret of the popular techniques of affirmation. It also applies to objects. The more we use, think about or wear a loved object on our bodies the more of our personal energy this object absorbs. With this technique it is the energy of the owner which has become part of the object that we connect with.

What Works? What Doesn't?

This technique is not for the professional private detective. It functions well with our own objects or those of our relatives. Perhaps a clairvoyant individual could use it for others as well but this is not my field.

Experiences	One of my students has had a lot of success with this technique finding all kinds of lost belongings, but I haven't lost anything in a long time so I am looking forward to the next time it happens!!!

Meditation with Rainbow Reiki

Prerequisite:
1st Reiki Degree

Technical Instructions

Step 1: Sit down comfortably with an erect spine and an upright pelvis. Hold your head as if your crown were being pulled gently up into the sky.

Step 2: Place the palms of your hands together in front of your heart. If you wish you can also place the soles of your feet together in the same way. In a variation of this exercise, you can place tumbled quartz crystals, fluorite, amethysts, rose

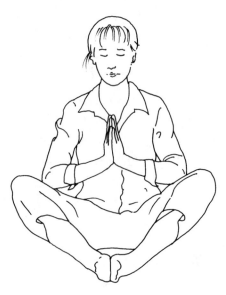

Opening

quartz or other healing stones of your choice between your palms and the soles of your feet. Reiki will stimulate the stones to radiate stronger healing energies. At the same time they support the body's receptivity to the pleasant vibrations of Reiki.

If you have been initiated you can also use the power symbol of the 2nd Degree between your palms and between the soles of your feet.

Length   15 minutes to more than 1 hour.

Please Note   Although less than 15 minutes of the Reiki meditation can promote relaxation, a deeper-reaching harmonization is usually not noticed in such a short time. The meditation should be done in a room with a pleasant temperature and should be uninterrupted.

Use   Consciousness expansion, spiritual experiences, deep relaxation, support of all types of healing processes, promotion of the ability to concentrate and learn, pain-relieving effects and the alleviation of psychosomatic complaints sometimes become possible.

Combination   Reiki for the Inner Child and the Higher Self, Reiki contact with angels and other spiritual beings, mental healing, crystal work, light-body work, mystic symbol practice with Rainbow Reiki.

Philosophy   With the help of meditation the mind can relax and the body shifts more easily into the state that is necessary for healing, regeneration and assimilation on all levels. Through meditative experiences an increasing degree of selfperception occurs and frequently a deep clearing of fears, fixations and limiting value judgments happens. In its many forms meditation has been used since the beginning of time for focused personality development and the support of healing processes. More deeply and addressed daily, the Buddhas have universally advised us that meditation leads to ultimate liberation.

What Works? What Doesn't?

Meditation works best when done as a regular daily practice. Over time there may be a profound harmonization and expansion of spiritual consciousness. It does not always immediately have a relaxing effect. Suppressed experience and emotions can rise up into the waking consciousness, needing to be integrated or acted out.

Experiences The Rainbow Reiki meditation is very well suited to people with a hectic daily routine. It is very good for those who want to learn to rest within themselves and do something for their health at the same time. I often recommend this exercise to stressed managers and clients who are going through particularly difficult crises in their life. It has worked well for them.

For a person who carries many suppressed feelings and a burdened subconscious mind some counseling and other Reiki exercises will be necessary along with the first sessions. Try mental healing and systematic chakra work in order to integrate or release these contents as they come up.

Meditation with the Distance-Treatment Symbol

Prerequisite:

2nd Reiki Degree

Technical Instructions

Step 1: Sit down undisturbed in a comfortable position for as long as you want. It is helpful to sit in full or half-lotus position but not absolutely necessary. Relax as much as possible and take a few deep breaths.

Step 2: Draw the distance-treatment symbol in the way that you like best and then mentally say the corresponding Mantra three times.

Step 3: Now repeat the name of the person, the place, or the situation with which you would like to connect during the meditation. This can be the name of your spiritual master, the name of a holy place or a specific consecrated situation.

Step 4: Say: "With the help of the Reiki symbol for the duration of this meditation I connect with … (name of person/place/situation.)"

Step 5: Then draw the mental-healing symbol and envelop the person/place/situation and yourself together in it.

Step 6: Seal everything with the power symbol, draw it once and repeat the Mantra three times.

Here is a variation of the meditation that I have practiced for many years:

Step 1: Sit down in a quiet place and close your eyes.

Step 2: Through the distance-treatment symbol connect yourself with this moment saying: "With the help of the Reiki symbol during this meditation I connect with the Here and Now."

Step 3: Now draw the mental-healing symbol once repeat the Mantra three times and wrap yourself in it.

Step 4: Seal everything with the power symbol, draw it once repeating the Mantra three times.

During the meditation if you notice that you are drifting off into your world of thoughts connect

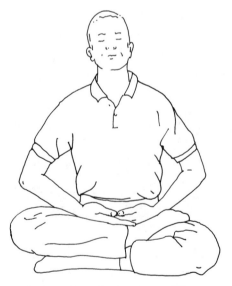

The heart beats in the Here and Now

once again with the Here and Now as described above.

Length 15-60 minutes.

Please Note It is necessary to rest afterwards. Right after the meditation you shouldn't drive or do any risky work that asks for your complete concentration. Take at least 15 minutes after the meditation before you again immerse yourself in the 'seriousness of life'.

Use With this technique you can connect with any person, any place or any situation that may deepen your meditation.

Combination It can be combined with meditation with the Reiki Master symbol as well as with any other type of meditation technique.

Philosophy Working alone on ourselves is not easy. Most spiritual teachers suggest that it is simply impossible and I suspect they could be right about this …. Using this technique we can connect with one who has arrived where we would like to be in the hope that their spark may flash across to ignite us. In my experience this works like a charm. Many of us have this experience: We sit down and within a few minutes all hell breaks loose in our minds. One thought chases the other like Tarzan and his band of chimps. With the help of this technique we can stop the craziness before it even starts!

What Works? What Doesn't?

This technique can help in connecting with the manifested light. Of course in a deeper sense all techniques are artificial and our ultimate goal in meditation, if you can call it a goal, consists of being meditative at all times, in every situation. And to be thus present without any crutches (techniques). No technique can replace the spiritual master.

Experiences After the death of my spiritual master Osho I stayed connected with him for many years by means of this technique. In actual fact this was not really necessary since the relationship to the master always remains intact, as is the bond to the parents. But it helped me through the times of uncertainty. Today I inhale and exhale my parents and my master with every breath ....

Meditation with the Master Symbol

Prerequisite:

3rd Reiki Degree

Technical Instructions

Step 1: Sit down undisturbed in a comfortable position for as long as suits you. It is helpful to sit in the full or half-lotus position but not absolutely necessary.

Step 2: Take a few deep breaths and with your dominant hand draw the Reiki Master symbol as large as possible in the air above your crown chakra. Then mentally say the corresponding Mantra three times.

Step 3: Stretch your arms above your head as straight as possible to the heavens and fold your hands, palms together, above your crown chakra.

Step 4: Stay in this position for a moment and then let both arms glide down at the same time in slow motion about 8 inches to the left and right of your head. As you do this imagine that you are putting the Master symbol into your aura. Continue with this until your arms are all the way down with the fingertips outstretched and pointing toward the earth.

Step 5: Now sit for the length of time you have set aside. Meditation should not be torture, it is a joy. Even five minutes just for yourself can give your day a whole new quality. If in the beginning it is difficult for you to sit be patient and let your body determine how long you dedicate to the meditation. After a few months it will probably be easy for you to sit for 30 or even 60 minutes without becoming bored or restless!

Length   5 to 60 minutes longer if possible.

Please Note   It is good to rest afterwards. Right after the meditation you should not drive or do any risky work that calls for concentration. Take at least 15 minutes before immersing yourself again in the 'seriousness of life'.

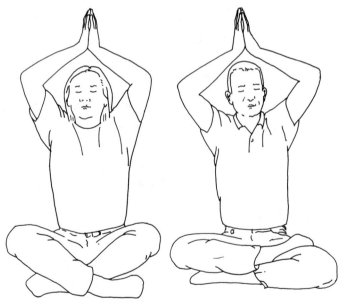

Imagine that you are absorbing the Master symbol into your aura

Use By using this method you can again feel connected with the cosmic energy source in just a few minutes. After practicing it for a while for many people meditation becomes a need, rather like spiritual food.

This technique is not however limited to silent meditation. You can apply it as often as you like and in every life situation. It's not even necessary to sit down to do this.

A friend of mine who is a great musical success in Japan always uses this technique before she goes on stage. And the audience loves her more and more ....

Combination Meditation techniques of the 2nd Reiki Degree, distant healing treatment (you send the Master symbol to a client or to yourself).

Philosophy The ego is a shadow entity, a dream. The moment we shine the light of the Master symbol on it we can, at least temporarily, awaken from this dream. The divine light is already within us and using the Master symbol simply activates or brings it into consciousness.

What Works? What Doesn't?

As already indicated in other places we cannot turn off the inner dialog with the help of a meditation technique. What we can however do with the help of a technique is create distance between ourselves and the constant chatter in our minds. As soon as we become aware of this we see that we and our inner dialog are two different things. And this is where the work really begins. Who are we, if we are not our thoughts, our feelings, our body ...?

The only meaningful question becomes: "Who am I?"

Experiences Many people know this experience:
The moment we sit down to meditate the inner dialog seems to really thrive. The more we then try to meditate the more difficult it becomes. With the Master symbol we can quickly become immersed in the most beautiful light. If we feel the inner dialog surging up in our mind, we redraw the Master symbol and are illuminated by its light once again.

I have done this meditation every day for years and can recommend it from the depths of my heart. It will bring you closer to yourself, to the light.

Mental Healing with Rainbow Reiki

Prerequisite:

2nd Reiki Degree

Technical Instructions

> *Step 1:* Place the left hand (if you are right-handed, otherwise use the right) on the back of the client's head.

> *Step 2:* With the right hand draw a mental-healing symbol on the crown of the head. Then repeat the corresponding Mantra three times while you hold the palm of your hand facing down onto the crown.

> *Step 3:* With the same hand draw a power symbol horizontally on the crown of the head. Place the hand on the crown and repeat the Mantra three times.

> *Step 4:* While both hands remain in the positions described above repeat three times the first and last name of the client or your own name if you are treating yourself.

> *Step 5:* After the contact has been established additional power symbols can be put on these positions.

> *Step 6:* Optionally the practitioner may mentally repeat a selected affirmation during the entire length of the treatment.

Step 7: End the mental healing by simply withdrawing your hands from the positions. It is not necessary to take leave since no distance contact has been created.

Length
5 to 10 minutes but considerably longer for greater problems. Using this technique Dr. Chujiro Hayashi treated people for up to 30 minutes per session.

Please Note
In many cases it is important to attach several power symbols to the back of the head in order to harmonize blocks in the cervical spine. These block the transmission of healing influences to the major and secondary chakras. If specific prob-

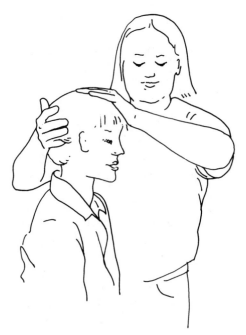

The hand position for Rainbow Reiki mental healing

lems are being treated instead of just a general promoting of personal development the use of appropriate affirmations is recommended. This can be worked out consciously or an appropriate question may be selected intuitively with the help of the *Chakra Energy Cards.*

Use   Change of problematic habits, addictions, fears, neurotic structures and complexes, psychosomatic complaints, support for spiritual development, integration of disassociated, partial personalities, life in the Here and Now.

Combination   KarmaClearing, systematic chakra work, Reiki for the Inner Child and the Higher Self.

Philosophy   Mental healing works directly on that part of the mind where all types of habitual patterns and routine behavior are formed and stored. Mental healing does not affect suggestion, programming or hypnosis. Affirmations only support Reiki in specific effects. Reiki itself always organizes the behavior programs in such a way that liveliness, health and happiness are promoted. Negative effects are not possible.

What Works? What Doesn't?

A lasting change in habits is only possible when the concerned person makes a conscious decision to continue on a new, healthier and more positive path. A lack of personal responsibility, postponement of decisions and a refusal to create and try out constructive alternatives to the old behavior patterns prevent a lasting change in destructive types of behavior. But with corresponding willingness even stubborn problems can be resolved in a gentle and enduring way. Mental healing is one of the most important Reiki techniques of all.

Experiences

Applying the mental healing technique I was once able to provide substantial help to a young woman who, as a result of an accident, suffered intense fear and recurring nightmares. In addition to individually selected affirmations I also used the help of regular energy balancing. This input works together with mental healing like Bach Flower Rescue Remedy.

Mystic Symbol Practice with Rainbow Reiki

Prerequisite:

2nd Reiki Degree (using the symbols and Mantras of the 2nd Degree)

3rd Reiki Degree (using the Master symbol)

Technical Instructions

Step 1: Select one of the symbols of the 2nd Degree or the Master symbol for the exercise.

Step 2: Hold both hands at chest height in front of your body with the palms facing forward.

Step 3: Now slowly, as if in slow motion, use the hand that you also write with to draw the symbol vertically in the air in front of you. It should be at least half as large as you are.

Step 4: When you have finished drawing the symbol hold your hands as explained in Step 2 and sing the Mantra associated with this symbol three times aloud and with a resonant voice.

Step 5: Slowly and consciously walk forward until you stand on the spot where you drew the symbol.

Step 6: Now put your legs close together and raise your arms to the sky, spreading them into the shape of a V. The palms should also be facing upward.

Alternative: Place your legs at about shoulder-width with feet parallel to each other. The legs should be slightly bent but the pelvis and the spinal column must be particularly straight. Hold your head as if there was a string attached to the crown that is gently pulling it upward.

Step 7: Remain in this position and breath into your hara an energy organ that is located approximately two fingerwidths below the navel on the midline of the body and about three fingerwidths into the pelvis.

Step 8: To close the exercise place your hands together in front of your heart, bow and give thanks. While bowing, raise your hands to your forehead in such a way that the tips of your index fingers touch the 6th chakra, a little above the bridge of the nose.

Step 9: Take a step back to the place where you stood at the beginning of the exercise. Take a few deep breaths and have a good stretch.

Length   Between 5 minutes and 1 hour depending upon how deep you want the spiritual experience to go.

Please Note   Immediately after the exercise don't operate heavy machinery, drive a car or do anything else that calls for full attention. It may take up to an hour but usually only about 15 minutes before the state of spiritual consciousness produced here gives way to that of everyday life. Grounding exercises can be helpful in returning to the material reality more quickly.

Use	The mystic symbol practice promotes the development of the spiritual self. Also with time it can give us deep insights and inspirations on the use of the Reiki symbols and their Mantras. This exercise can also support the harmonization of mental-emotional problems.
Combination	Contact with the Higher Self and the Inner Child, contact with angels and other spiritual beings, light-body work with Rainbow Reiki.
Philosophy	Through the very slow, attentive drawing of a symbol and the singing of its Mantra a very strong energy structure is built through which the practitioner can directly experience the spiritual quality of the symbol in the meditation. This serves to develop the spiritual qualities represented by the symbol within the individual. In some cases it may also have a positive influence on health disorders. The results of the exercise depend on the regularity and attention with which we practice it.

What Works? What Doesn't?

Practicing this technique regularly creates a deep intuitive access to the protective spirit of the Reiki system. In Japanese Shingon (esoteric Buddhism) this is called the transcendent Buddha, *Dainichi Nyorai* who is the great radiant light from which all spiritual powers flow.

Experiences	People who have used this exercise daily over an extended period almost always report sensations of deep unity or spiritual inspiration. For me the mystic symbol practice is an important exercise

that helps me to be open to places of power and to maintain a spiritual perspective on my decisions when things get hectic.

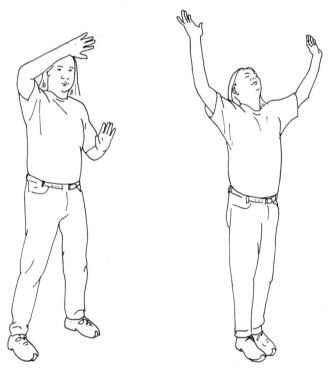

A) Draw the symbol (left)
B) Stand in the symbol and feel the spiritual power (right—both hands up)

Objects—Treating with Reiki

Prerequisite:

1st Reiki Degree

Technical Instructions

Step 1: Sit down comfortably and take a few deep breaths.

Step 2: Enclose the object to be treated in your hands.

Step 3: Now let the energy flow for at least five minutes. Follow your feelings as to the length of the treatment. If you sense a tingling, a magnetic feeling or an unusual amount of heat or cold in your hands treat the object until this feeling disappears.

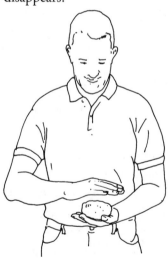

A Reiki treatment even lends wings to a stone

If you have mastered the 2ⁿᵈ Reiki Degree you can now let the symbols flow. The basic rules for this are:

• Use the distance-treatment symbol to establish contact with an object.

• To strengthen an object use the power symbol.

• To harmonize it use the mental-healing symbol.

If the object to be treated does not fit into your hands place them upon it. If it is too large for this or is located at another place use the techniques of the distant healing treatment with the 2ⁿᵈ Reiki Degree.

Length   5 to 15 minutes.

Please Note   I used to think that illness and dangerous external influences could be avoided through a pure heart. But unfortunately this is not the case. Avoid touching any type of radioactive material!

Use   This technique is used to charge objects with Reiki.

Combination   Distant healing treatment.

Philosophy   Everything in our world responds to energy. People, animals and plants are the most receptive but other things also react to Reiki treatment. Cars, computers and batteries can often be treated or charged successfully.
Even mundane things like two glasses stuck inside each other can be treated with Reiki so that you can separate them.

What Works? What Doesn't?

A shattered teacup will not be repaired with Reiki. But the tea that we drink from any cup will taste better. If the cup has but a crack it is possible to prolong its life with Reiki. But even a teacup is not immortal.

Experiences
During a Reiki group two glasses had become stuck inside each other in the sink. No one was able to separate them so tightly were they joined. I used the opportunity to demonstrate the gentle power of Reiki. Holding the glasses in my hands for a few seconds they were immediately freed from each other. I still laugh about this story since one of the participants was convinced that I had pulled a trick on her to win her over to Reiki!

Parking Space—Looking for with Reiki

Prerequisite:

2nd Reiki Degree

Technical Instructions

You can use this technique either before or while driving a car.

Step 1: Take a few deep breaths and draw the power symbol once. Mentally repeat its Mantra three times strongly.

Step 2: Say three times: "I will find a good parking space, parking space, parking space in such and such location …."

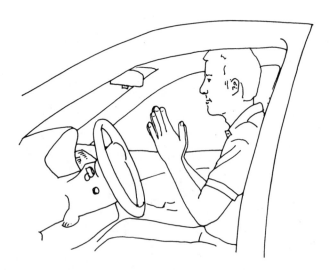

It's best to use this technique before you drive

Step 3: Drive to your destination completely relaxed.

Using the power symbol you can also change the
traffic signals to green!

Length	2 minutes.
Please Note	Using Reiki in traffic does not protect you from recklessness. So always be careful and loving whenever you are behind the wheel. If you are upset, work on this before you drive off or let someone else drive. ("Emotional Problems— Treating with Reiki," see page 152.)
Use	This technique is used to find a parking space peacefully.
Combination	Distant healing treatment for situations in the future, affirmation technique.
Philosophy	The art of sending energy successfully depends on our powers of concentration. When we are capable of concentrating our mind and our thoughts we can influence the world around us. Nothing in this world is free, without some effort of our own. We have always to give in order to get something in return.

This rule should kept in mind when we work
with a Reiki technique to actualize a personal
wish. Reiki is intended for the good of the whole
but this does not mean that it won't work when
we use it for our personal profit. We should always look carefully at the motives behind our
own wishes.

What Works? What Doesn't?

Trust is good but it doesn't replace our responsibility to use common sense. Rather than drive to the soccer stadium it might be better to use public transport.

Experiences Many Reiki friends use this technique in the big cities of the world. I have experienced how it is possible to find parking spaces in Paris, London, or Mexico City at the most difficult times of the day. And precisely where they were needed! Personally though I prefer to drift with the current of the present moment.

Plant Communication with Reiki

Prerequisite:

2nd Reiki Degree

Technical Instructions

Step 1: Sit or stand relaxed and take in several deep breaths.

Step 2: Draw the distance-treatment symbol once in the way most comfortable for you and repeat the corresponding Mantra mentally three times.

Step 3: Then say the name, the term for the plant or garden, the field or the forest to be treated.

Step 4: Now say: "I would like to speak with the consciousness of the plant …."

Step 5: Ask what is wrong with the plant and whether it may have any type of request. Be all ears!

Step 6: Then draw the mental-healing symbol once, repeat the Mantra three times and mentally place the symbol on the plant. Wish it peace and harmony.

Step 7: Close the 'conversation with the plant' by using the power symbol (draw it once and repeat the Mantra three times).

Length

5 to 10 minutes. If necessary use repeatedly over a longer period of time.

Please Note   If there is a strong pest or fungus infection all of the love in the world won't help. Take action as quickly as possible. Ask a specialist about possible organic remedies.

Use   This technique can help you to connect with plants, gardens, fields and forests.

Combination   Plants—Treatment with 1st Reiki Degree, distant healing treatment (send distance Reiki to your plant or your entire garden, a field, a meadow or a forest).

Philosophy   As Dr. Mikao Usui said in the interview mentioned above (printed in *Reiki—The Legacy of Dr. Usui)*, the human being is the most highly developed living being on Earth. This state also brings with it specific responsibilities including that of caring for the well being of all other living beings on the Earth.

All living beings are connected on a level that usually remains hidden from us. The Reiki symbols can help us to establish contact with the consciousness of other beings and initiate any needed action.

What Works? What Doesn't?

I have often experienced a plant telling me what is wrong with it. Working with this technique we must listen to our intuition since, in the beginning, the plant may be quite timid and modest in its messages. Don't doubt yourself when an inner voice says that a plant would like to move to some other location. It has no legs, so the life force has engaged you for this purpose.

And this is good way to see yourself: as a being in the service of the life force.

Experiences Some years ago I had a beautiful plant in my office which was threatening to give up the ghost despite the good care that I give all of my potted plants. After a few days it turned yellow and sullenly let all its leaves hang down. I had almost given up hope. As I was in the process of repotting it I asked what was wrong and how I could help. A silent dialog sprang up between us and it seemed that the plant wanted to move to a specific spot in another room. I fulfilled this request immediately and within a few days it was more beautiful and healthy than ever.

Plants—Treating with Reiki 1

Prerequisite:

1st Reiki Degree

Technical Instructions

Put your hands around the plant or its pot and let the energy flow for a few minutes.

The same rules apply as for treating a living person. When you have placed your hands in a position where the energy is being strongly absorbed you will feel a tingling or a magnetic sensation, heaviness or lightness, cold or warmth. Keep your hands in this position until they feel 'totally normal' again.

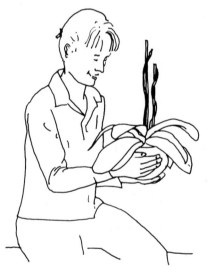

Hold the pot in your hands

If the plant is too large to grasp place both hands on its trunk or on the soil around it.

You can also enrich water that you give your plants with Reiki. Hold the watering can with both hands for 2 minutes and let the energy flow. Treat the water for 5 minutes when you plan to sprinkle it on a sick plant.

Length   5 to 15 minutes.

Please Note   To treat fungus infection or pest infestations you need to act quickly. There are many organic controls for fungus and pests. Let a specialist give you detailed advice on this.

Use   With the help of this technique you can provide your house and garden plants with Reiki. They will reward you with a great luxuriance of flowers and fruit!

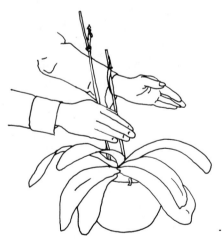

Or hold your hands above the plant

Combination   Plants—Treatment with the 2nd Reiki Degree, distant healing treatment—send distance Reiki to your plants or your entire garden, field, meadow or forest.

Philosophy   Plants feel just as people and animals do. It is no longer a secret that the growth of plants can be strongly influenced by music as well as by human love and attention. In turn healthy plants in our living spaces have positive effects on us human beings.

What Works? What Doesn't?

We can certainly make the life of our plants more pleasant for them. Reiki cannot however stop them from dying. Every living being dies when its time has come.

Experiences   Potted plants that I have never seen in bloom even in their tropical homelands are blossoming in my office. The plants in the room where I give Reiki initiations always flower ahead of other houseplants. The most surprising results came from several dracaena plants (massangeana, botanical name: dracaena fragrans). They had such a strong fragrance that for weeks the entire building was permeated with the sweetest perfume.

Plants—Treating with Reiki 2

Prerequisite:

2nd Reiki Degree

Technical Instructions

> *Step 1:* Draw the distance-treatment symbol once and mentally repeat the corresponding Mantra three times.

> *Step 2:* Now address the plants that you want to enrich with energy. Repeat their names or a short description three times (for example: 'the plant sitting on the bookshelf in my parents' living room').

> *Step 3:* Draw the mental-healing symbol once and repeat the Mantra three times.

> *Step 4:* Seal everything with the power symbol, draw it once and repeat the Mantra three times .

> *Step 5:* Now let the energy flow for a few minutes ....

If you place your hands on the plant to be treated put them around its trunk, a branch or its pot.
You can also enrich the water you give your plants with the Reiki symbol by writing it with your hand on the watering can or projecting it with your inner or outer eyes.
Hold the watering can for 2 minutes with both hands and let the symbols flow out of your hands into the water.

You can also give the entire garden a distant healing treatment (see pages 138-148).

Length	5 to 15 minutes.
Please Note	To treat fungus infection or pest infestations you must act quickly. There are many organic methods to control these. Let a specialist give you detailed advice.
Use	With the help of this technique you can provide your house and garden plants with Reiki or distance Reiki.
Combination	Plants—Treatment with the 1st Degree Reiki distant healing treatment, distant healing—treatment of situations in the future (blossoming, harvest or growth).
Philosophy	For more than 20 years there has been scientific evidence of the sentient life of plants as well as the existence of morphogenetic fields. These are invisible energy fields that connect the human, animal and plant worlds with each other. I believe that Reiki flows along this morphogenetic information highway between practitioner and recipient.

What Works? What Doesn't?

Plants in Reiki clinics or rooms where initiations take place always look great. Moreover our plants are as happy as children when their parents come home! In addition to energetic nourishment plants also need a beneficial location and good water, soil and compost.

Experiences	Friends of ours in Australia have been treating their paradise garden with 2nd Reiki Degree for years. It

has neither pests nor fungal infestation and the entire garden vibrates with the light of love and harmony. The neighbors whose gardens are attacked from all sides don't have a clue how they do it ....

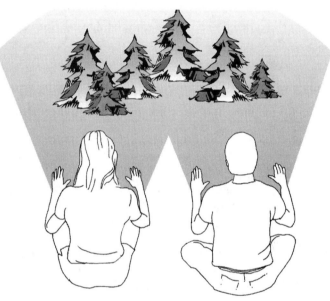

This is how you can improve your garden's microclimate

Protection Against Energy Vampires

Prerequisite:
2nd Reiki Degree

Technical Instructions

Step 1: As soon as you feel that your energy is being tapped by someone else or that you are being psychically attacked draw the power symbol once and mentally repeat the corresponding Mantra three times.

Step 2: Now let down a shield made of the power symbol between you and the source of the disturbance.

Step 3: Let go of your difficulties and the fear of losing energy or of a psychic attack.

Length 3 minutes, as soon as you notice that protection is diminishing begin over again.

Please Note In most cases a drop in our energy level is related to ourselves. Be careful not to project the responsibility for this onto others.

Use This technique can be used as protection against 'energy vampires' and psychic attacks. Garlic usually doesn't help.

Combination Distant healing treatment, grounding technique, distand healing treatment of situations in the future, whole body protection with the power symbol.

Philosophy   We have all certainly experienced this when visiting a sick person in hospital. It is as though ones life force is abruptly cut off, energy reserves are suddenly gone and one would like nothing more than to climb into the first available bed!

This can also happen in the presence of apparently healthy people. If you feel quickly drained and tired in the presence of a certain individual it may be a good idea to avoid contact with this person. If this is not possible you can use this technique:

Feeling other people's bad thoughts you must learn to not let them touch you. This is easily done by saying out loud: "This has nothing to do with me!"

What Works? What Doesn't?

This technique cannot help you through unpleasant situations because it is only a band-aid or a way to temporarily patch things up. The best 'protective measure' is simply to be ourselves and let anything negative that comes our way flow right through us. However we can use the protection technique described above until this has been mastered.

Experiences   In the beginning of my public Reiki work I felt quite frequently psychically attacked. This began three days after the publication of my first book and went on for several years. I was completely unprepared because I had assumed that my research on Dr. Mikao Usui and the actual history of Reiki would be received with great joy. Instead I received threats and the nastiest stories were spread about me. When I now look back at this time I do so with love.

Through these constant confrontations I have grown and learned to stand in my own light. I am very grateful to my attackers for this lesson. What can be learned from difficult situations is to be yourself and feel at home in every situation life presents. In truth you are always at home!

Protection with Reiki Against Emotional Injuries

Prerequisite:
2nd Reiki Degree

Technical Instructions

Step 1: Sit or stand comfortably and take a few deep breaths.

Step 2: Draw the mental-healing symbol once and mentally repeat the corresponding Mantra three times.

Step 3: Mentally place the symbol on your heart or the heart of the recipient and feel the energy.

Step 4: Seal everything with the power symbol (draw it once and repeat the Mantra three times).

Step 5: Concentrate on your heart area. Feel how your heart opens and how the heart chakra is activated and strengthened by the symbol.

Step 6: Let the energy flow ….

Length   5 to 10 minutes

Please Note   This technique can also be used as a distant healing treatment. As already mentioned you should have the permission of the recipient to do this. It is a good idea to rest afterwards. The recipient should not drive or do risky work that calls for concentration during or shortly after the session.

It may be important to talk to someone you trust after the treatment.

Use This technique can be used when you feel emotionally wounded.

Combination Distant healing treatment, also for yourself, whole-body treatment, affirmation technique.

Philosophy In its original form the mental-healing symbol represents the Amida Buddha, the Buddha of Love and Compassion at the Kurama Temple in Kyoto. By calling on this symbol we connect with a powerful patron of spiritual protection.

What Works? What Doesn't?

We can build up our emotional immune system with this technique. With a little bit of practice we can use it to free ourselves from the influence of emotional attacks. However even with the help of the Amida Buddha we cannot make others do what is best for them. So emotional attacks are not prevented via this technique but it helps us to deal with them in a better way.

The more sensitive we become the greater the suffering we are exposed to. However our openness to joy and happiness also grows to the same degree.

Experiences Since a friend started using this technique emotional injuries are no longer a problem for her. In the beginning she frequently used it and would ask me to back her up with it too. But now negative input no longer bothers her. The mental-healing symbol has completed its work!

Many people have observed that Reiki sometimes erases our obstructive behavior patterns and does it so gently that we don't even notice. A few years later it suddenly occurs to us: What happened to that anger, that jealousy, that fear?

Psychic Contact with Reiki

Prerequisite:
2nd Reiki Degree

When we have learned to center our thoughts this technique, which involves making contact with people and animals on a psychic level, works easily even without Reiki.

Technical Instructions

Step 1: Sit down as comfortably as possible in a place where you will not be disturbed for at least 15 minutes.

Step 2: Concentrate on the person or the animal you want to establish *contact with.*

Step 3: Draw the distance-treatment symbol once and repeat the corresponding Mantra three times.

Step 4: Mentally draw the distance-treatment symbol on the third eye of the person or the animal you want to reach.

Step 5: Say the name of the person or the animal three times.

Step 6: Concentrate on your third eye and say three times: "I hereby establish contact with ... (name the person or the animal)."

Step 7: Send your message to the person (the animal). For example when you want to reach your partner say: " ... (name of the person) call me as soon as possible," or: " ... (name of the person) come home as quickly as you can."

Step 8: Draw the mental-healing symbol once repeat the Mantra three times and send it to the person or animal.

Step 9: Seal everything with the power symbol, draw it once and say the Mantra three times.

Length 3 to 10 minutes.

Please Note This technique is intended for emergency situations. If you would like to experiment with it for fun do so only after discussing it with the person you are trying to reach and get their approval. You can arrange with them to call you on their mobile phone the moment they feel mental contact with you.

Use Using this technique you can psychically connect with any living being you may want to. It is mainly used for contacting people who for one reason or another cannot be reached. You can even call yourself with it if you have this problem!

Combination Distance Reiki treatment of people and animals, Comatose People—Treating with Reiki.

Philosophy When our attention is centered in the forehead, the third eye chakra, dream and the reality merge into one whole. This means that from this energy center we can manifest whatever we want to achieve. Once again there is a fine line between beauty and danger here.

What Works? What Doesn't?

Before using this technique on strangers it's best to experiment on someone from our immediate circle of friends or family. Our favorite actor certainly won't start feverishly looking for us if we connect with him in this way.

This is not a party trick and should only be used when sincerely needed. Sending unwanted messages is manipulation and absolutely not recommended.

Experiences

When my cat was about a year old it disappeared without a trace. I called it every few hours for several days and scoured the entire neighborhood. I had almost given up when I used this technique to send it the message that I would be going out soon to look for it again. I had the feeling that it might have crawled into an open garage and been inadvertently locked in.

Out in the street I called it and called it. This was about one o'clock in the morning. Then from nowhere I heard a muted 'meow' but couldn't figure where it was coming from. I called and called again and an answer came from the distance each time. Shining my flashlight on the neighboring houses suddenly I saw our cat standing in a second floor window! It had climbed in while the house was being cleaned and managed to get itself locked inside. The neighbors hadn't even noticed it yet ....

Rainbow Reiki for the Higher Self

Prerequisite:

2nd Reiki Degree

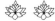

Technical Instructions

Step 1: Draw the distance-treatment symbol and say its Mantra quietly three times. Then draw the power symbol and also say its Mantra three times. Now turn your hands away from yourself and assume that wherever they point is where your Higher Self is located. But do not try to visualize this. If a mental picture arises this is fine but don't hold onto the image. It is not necessary to get a picture of your Higher Self for this technique to function. Speak to it three times with the words: "Higher Self of ... (add your own first and last names)."

Step 2: Use the power symbol with its Mantra several times in order to provide more Reiki. Pay attention to what is happening inside you: your body perception, your feelings and any images that may arise. If there is something you need to deal with ask the Higher Self for its help in working through current problem areas effectively. Otherwise ask it to stand by you on your path with advice and support. Don't expect any special attention during the contact. Ask it for messages that it thinks are important for you.

The effects of the work with your Higher Self will mostly show up later in your everyday life.

Step 3: Take leave with the words: "I take leave of you Higher Self of ... (adding your first and last names)." Blow vigorously between your hands and then rub the palms together.

Length
About 5 to 10 minutes once you have become accustomed to it. You can obviously also do it for longer. Even if you don't have much time for the exercise a brief contact is better than none at all. Don't expect anything specific from the contact so that anything and everything can happen.

Please Note
Right after the contact make a note of your experiences so that you don't forget anything important.

Use
For improving the quality of your life, to accompany all the difficulties in life, especially for chronic illnesses or problems for which you cannot find a solution, to promote spiritual development, to attract suitable friends, a partner and professional contacts, to have more happiness and good fortune.

Combination
Reiki for the Inner Child, distant healing treatment, contact treatment, chakra work, mental healing, contacts with angels.

Philosophy
The Higher Self is one of the three archetypal parts of every individual personality. The other two are the Middle Self and the Inner Child. The Higher Self of an individual is constantly involved in creating opportunities for learning in the spiritual sense. It makes the appropriate

contacts and generates the resources necessary for healthy self development. It allows for abundant happy 'coincidences' and prevents difficulties or makes them easier to harmonize.

However the Higher Self is not a 'magic lantern' to make our wishes all come true. The emphasis of its activities is the spiritual quality of our life and it needs energy in order to fulfil its tasks. Through the Reiki contact it is provided with power. Further possibilities for sending the Higher Self energy with which to carry out its duties are: sincere prayer, leading a spiritual life, good deeds, spiritual offerings and rituals that serve higher purposes.

What Works? What Doesn't?

Within the scope of its functions the Higher Self can accomplish many things. It cannot however be used by the Middle Self, the everyday consciousness, to serve *its* purpose. Only when a request of the Middle Self is spiritually meaningful will the Higher Self go to work on its behalf. A certain amount of time is often necessary before the Higher Self of an individual has gathered enough energy to become active again after fulfilling a task.

Experiences When I began to work with this technique absolutely nothing happened for about three months. Then positive events followed in quick succession. I suddenly received a lot of unexpected support in my search for suitable seminar rooms, my first book was published and I was invited to work both at home and abroad.

Rainbow Reiki for the Inner Child

Prerequisite:

2nd Reiki Degree

Technical Instructions

> *Step 1:* Draw the distance-treatment symbol and quietly say its Mantra three times. Then draw the power symbol and also say its Mantra three times. Turn your hands away from yourself and assume that where they are pointing is where your Inner Child is located. But do not visualize it. Speak to it three times with the words: "Inner Child of … (add your first and last names)."

> *Step 2:* Use the power symbol with its Mantra several times to provide more Reiki. Pay attention to what is happening inside you. Ask your Inner Child for its help in effectively working through current problems. Don't expect any special attention, the effects of the work with the Inner Child will show up later in your daily life rather than during the contact. Ask it for information that it thinks important for you and be open for any form in which the answer may come, like body sensations, moods, images, etc. Ask what you can do for its well-being. Ask it to be more available to you in your everyday life. If you have no specific issues simply feel your way into the contact and enjoy a deep sense of connectedness with your Inner Child.

Step 3: Take leave with the words: "I take leave of you, Inner Child of ... (add your first and last names)." Blow vigorously between your hands and then rub the palms together.

Length

About 5 to 10 minutes once you have become accustomed to it. You can obviously also do it for longer. Even if you don't have much time for the session a brief contact is better than none at all.

Please Note

Right after the contact make a note of your experiences so that you don't forget anything important. Don't expect anything in particular from the experience so that anything and everything can happen.

Use

Promoting intuition, body consciousness and healing processes of all types, very effective as a supporting treatment for all kinds of problems associated with the first two major chakras.

Combination

Reiki for the Higher Self, distant healing treatment, contact treatment, chakra work, mental healing, bodywork with Reiki.

Philosophy

The Inner Child is one of the three archetypal parts of every individual's personality. The other two are the Middle Self and the Higher Self. By giving Reiki to the Inner Child its connection to the other two archetypal parts of the personality is improved and stabilized, and its development and the scope of its action are promoted.

What Works? What Doesn't?

Reiki for the Inner Child supports joy, playfulness, fun and a positive attitude toward the body and its needs. It is however also important to maintain a lifestyle that corresponds.

Experiences

A psychiatrist friend of mine asked me to give Reiki to a patient with an acute psychosis. This was in addition to his on going therapy. After meditating, 'Reiki for the Inner Child' occurred to me as the best technique for her. Because the case was very acute I gave Reiki to her Inner Child for several hours each day. Two days later her state was already much calmer. After a week she was able to leave the psychiatric ward and go onto a lower dose of her medication.

Reiki Alarm Clock

Prerequisite:

2nd Reiki Degree

Technical Instructions

> *Step 1:* Draw the distance-treatment symbol once and mentally repeat the corresponding Mantra three times.

> *Step 2:* Say your own name at the beginning: " ... please wake up at 6:30 a.m. well-rested and in a good mood."

> *Step 3:* Draw the mental-healing symbol once and say the Mantra three times.

> *Step 4:* Seal everything with the power symbol (draw it once and repeat the Mantra three times).

> *Step 5:* Good night!

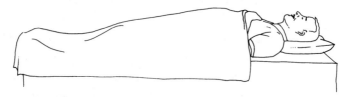

It works best if you use this practice just before falling asleep

Length   3 to 5 minutes.

Please Note   Reiki does not turn you into Superman or Superwoman. Adequate sleep is the basis of an alert life.

Use This technique can help you wake up without an alarm clock at a specific time feeling well-rested.

Combination Whole-body treatment before going to sleep, distant healing treatment for situations in the future, deprogramming.

Philosophy The subconscious mind is an unfamiliar aspect of our existence. But it is a large part of life and we can learn to draw strength from it. When this is achieved with a simple technique like the one described here it releases enormous powers. We notice that we have much more in reserve and that our capacities and our possibilities are far from exhausted. This provides us with a great boost.

What Works? What Doesn't?

Using this technique we can literally wake ourselves up. I have never tried it on another person and I suspect that it would not be helpful. We must always ask ourselves whether a technique is beneficial for the growth of the person who practices it and for whoever is being treated. If this is not the case then it is missing its mark.

If for example a child does not wake up in the morning because he doesn't want to go to school, it would be advisable to look at the basic problem before trying Reiki to alleviate the symptom.

Experiences For some years now I have been travelling a great deal and frequently need to get up early or appear at some gray airport at an ungodly hour. Since childhood I have been allergic to alarm clocks. This expresses itself in several ways. I either turn it off in the beginning, set it incorrectly from the start or even forget to pack it in the first place. Right now I am sitting here in Mexico City without an alarm clock. However with the help of this technique I always wake up before my alarm clock would go off when I do have one set nicely, *and* with enough time to turn it off. So my allergy is taken care of—by Reiki!

After some experience with this exercise you probably won't need to use the symbols any more. You simply call yourself by name and ask that you wake up well-rested, in a good mood at a specific time.

Reiki Box

Prerequisite:
2ⁿᵈ Reiki Degree

Technical Instructions

1ˢᵗ Phase:

> *Step 1:* Take a closeable wooden or cardboard box that is large enough to hold several sheets of paper.
>
> *Step 2:* Write the name, the object or the situation that you would like to treat, or an affirmation etc on a sheet of paper. This can include several pieces of paper.
>
> *Step 3:* Draw the distance-treatment symbol on the page and mentally repeat the corresponding Mantra three times.
>
> *Step 4:* Then repeat three times the name of your client, the situation, the name of the place etc. that you would like to treat.
>
> *Step 5:* Draw the mental-healing symbol on the page and repeat the Mantra three times.
>
> *Step 6:* Stabilize everything with the power symbol, draw it once and repeat the Mantra three times.

Step 7: Place your hands on the piece of paper and let the energy flow for a few minutes, for as long as it feels good, 5 to 10 minutes are certain to be enough.

Step 8: Put the written page or pages in the box and close it.

2nd Phase:

Step 1: Draw the distance-treatment symbol directly on the box and say: "With the help of the Reiki symbol please give as much energy for as long as it is required for the greatest good of everyone involved in this situation."

Step 2: Now draw the mental-healing symbol once on the box and repeat the Mantra three times.

Step 3: Stabilize everything with the power symbol which you draw once repeating the Mantra three times.

Step 4: Let the energy flow for a few minutes.

Repeat both phases everyday for at least a week. If you want to treat the box for an additional week start over from the beginning again.

Length
According to the number of clients or situations to be treated, 5 to 15 minutes or even longer if necessary.

Please Note
If you use the Reiki box to treat other people, as applies to all techniques of the distant healing treatment, you should have the permission of the recipient beforehand.

Use   This technique can help you in sending Reiki simultaneously to several people or situations.

Combination   Affirmation technique, distant healing treatment, deprogramming.

Philosophy   In terms of the energy needed it doesn't matter whether we send Reiki to one person or several people or situations at the same time. Reiki energy penetrates the entire universe and can therefore be sent from an initiate to any recipients anywhere.

What Works? What Doesn't?

This technique is designed for working with several clients at the same time. We need however to be sure that we do not overextend ourselves or lose contact with our client. So put down the

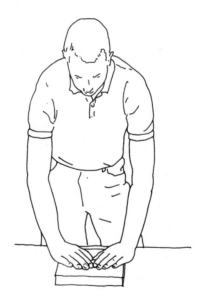

This is how you can treat several people or situations at the same time

telephone book and begin by experimenting with a short list!

Experiences When I was starting out with Reiki I used this technique every day. At that time I was not happy with many aspects of my life in both the material world and my own inner process. Over the years this technique has helped me build my self-assurance and self-confidence to a point where I noticed that I no longer needed the technique. But this is the second step which comes well after the first, so enjoy working with this exercise!

Reiki Shower with Rainbow Reiki

Prerequisite:

2nd Reiki Degree

Technical Instructions

Step 1: In the vicinity of the spot where you want the Reiki shower to work place a distance-treatment symbol and activate it by saying or thinking its Mantra three times.

Step 2: Draw one or more power symbols over the place where you want the Reiki shower. The more power symbols you apply the stronger the effect will be. When you do this the symbols must be drawn in such a way that one flat side faces the distance-treatment symbol and the other flat

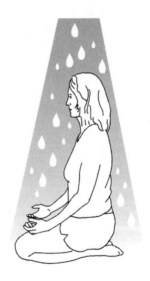

side faces the place to which you want the Reiki to flow. Activate each symbol with its Mantra three times.

Length

A Rainbow Reiki shower can be applied for a given period as a limited measure such as intensifying a Reiki or massage session. It can also be used as an energy enhancement that is meant to last. A Reiki shower will diminish in its effects over time until at some point it completely disappears. But once it has been created it cannot be simply 'switched off'. The duration of the effect ranges from about 20 minutes under very difficult conditions to several days under the best. How long it lasts depends on certain prevailing factors: the attention and serious-mindedness of the creation of the Reiki shower itself, disharmonious Feng Shui in the room, the number of people using the room and how they harmonize emotionally with each other, the intensity of electrical and other disruptive radiation, construction materials and so on.

Because some of the conditions can never be predicted I have discovered that the only real away to control these effects is to use my intuition, my subtle perception in the moment to read the environment.

Please Note

It is useful to take time before and after creating a Reiki shower to feel the quality and strength of the energy in the room in that moment. This is an easy way to develop your powers of subtle perception. Through feeling directly it is also the easiest way to determine whether a room needs to be

Reiki Shower with Rainbow Reiki

255

cleansed or if the energetic situation is still positive.

Create a Reiki shower for others only with their express permission.

Use

With the Rainbow Reiki shower we can build a long-lasting, localized Reiki field in a specific place requiring no additional energy work or attention to maintain it. This means that once built the Reiki shower does its work without anyone needing to attend to it.

This is a very practical technique. You can use it to Reiki- charge a (hotel) bed, the seats in your car or a place that is subjected to disharmonious earth radiation. Through the years the Reiki shower has proved to be very helpful in dozens of situations. Consider this list: Creation of personal power spots, promotion of plant growth and pest remedies, sending patients an 'extra boost' of Reiki in addition to actual treatments, for energetic cleansing and the positive charging of jewelry, healing stones and card sets (for a thorough cleansing and charging, please reckon with 4 to 8 hours of influence time … the more regularly something is placed under the Reiki shower the less influence time it needs), to make Reiki healing water from normal water (please use non-carbonated water because the gas bubbles of carbonation carry Reiki out of the water fast, and place it under the Reiki shower for about 6 to 8 hours), to energize drinks and foods, to create a positive atmosphere at the workplace, to render chemical medications more tolerable, creating additional positive influences during Reiki sessions, massages, acupuncture treatments, psychotherapeutic or healing-stone sessions, etc. With some practice in visualization the Rainbow Reiki shower can also be applied via the Reiki distant healing treatment. With a little creativity you can easily find many more ways to use this simple, very effective and flexible Reiki tool in your every day life.

Combination Among other things: Rainbow Reiki room cleansing, whole-body treatment, Rainbow Reiki meditation, mental healing with Rainbow Reiki, candle ritual with Rainbow Reiki, crystal fountains with Rainbow Reiki .

Philosophy Via the distance-treatment symbol a lasting Reiki source continuing to exist even without added distance-treatment contact or any other measures is established close to the place where the Rainbow Reiki shower is needed. Using the power symbol the latent Reiki existing in the distance-treatment symbol is drawn to the chosen area of activity.

Please be absolutely sure to note this: In order for the Rainbow Reiki shower to function as described the power symbol must be drawn moving in a counterclockwise direction.

What Works? What Doesn't?

Problematic environmental conditions can be harmonized up to a point. However in cases involving major problems of disruptive radiation and bad Feng Shui it is always better to work directly on the causes of the imbalances. As effective as the Rainbow Reiki shower may be it can only support individual contact or distant healing treatment, not replace it.

Experiences　One of my Reiki students had an interesting experience with her dog, a large Golden Retriever. Once when it had digestive problems the animal lay down directly under the Reiki shower that she had created above her meditation space. The dog had never sought out this place before. He quickly went to sleep there.

Later when the Reiki shower had not been renewed for three days because of a visiting relative, the dog walked confusedly around the spot as if looking for something. As soon as the Reiki shower was created again he was content to lie down and soon fell asleep right on the spot.

Room—Cleansing with Rainbow Reiki

Prerequisite:

2nd Reiki Degree

Technical Instructions

Step 1: Draw the distance-treatment symbol at a place in the room where you can see as many of its corners as possible. This is usually somewhere in the center of the room. Say the corresponding Mantra quietly three times.

Step 2: In each of the corners of the room visible from the distance-treatment symbol draw at least one power symbol and say its Mantra three times. The power symbols should have one flat side pointing to the corner and the other side facing the distance-treatment symbol in the center of the room. This is the only way they can develop their full power of harmonization. If there are protruding edges on the walls or large pieces of furniture these should also have the power symbol attached to them in the same way.

Length

Depending on the energetic environmental influences the time needed to cleanse a room varies. Train your abilities of subtle perception regularly by checking before and after a room cleansing to see how you feel there. Does the space feel tight or open? Cold or warm? Does it flow around you or does it stand still? Do you feel heavy or light? This way you can easily tell whether a room needs cleansing or not. It is very like a searching look into the kitchen to see if it's time to do the dishes and clean up again.

Please Note   If there are many nooks and corners, large pieces of furniture and small plants in the room this cleansing will be more complicated. It means that you need to attach several power symbols per corner or edge and actually attend to each one of them.

Use   Energetic cleansing of rooms, Feng Shui, increasing the spiritual vibration of rooms, creating an atmosphere that supports healing, promoting the growth and health of plants, creating a power place within a building, clearing and harmonizing the room energies after healing sessions, consultations, seminars and rituals, or interpersonal conflicts.

Combination   Reiki shower, Reiki for the Higher Self of a house, Reiki for the Inner Child of a house, Karma-Clearing for a building.

Philosophy   Energies that cannot flow tend to collect in the corners of a room and this is why the Reiki symbols are directed there. A cleansing with Reiki restores the natural, life-promoting flow of energy in a room. It does not directly remove anything. Flowing, vital energy always promotes life while congested life energy reduces vitality creating a sense of dis-ease, disharmonious moods, nervousness and irritability, encouraging the development of health problems.

According to the Chinese teaching of Feng Shui edges pointing into a room even radiate the so-called *sha.* This is a concentric energy form that moves in straight lines. Its effect on human beings, animals and most plants is like a cold draft. With the Reiki technique of room-cleansing this disharmony can be cancelled out.

What Works? What Doesn't?

Room-cleansing alone is not enough when a building has been through very difficult and traumatic times. When vehement conflicts, long and serious illnesses, crimes or even murder or suicide have taken place the other techniques mentioned above should be used as well. If the room has furnishings connected with situations traumatic for its inhabitants it is worth making a thorough attempt to harmonize these objects energetically. However in order to restore a tolerable atmosphere furnishings often have to be removed.

Experiences   On a trip once I arrived one evening at a little hotel in Provence. I was in a good mood but as soon as I had settled into my clean, cozy room for no apparent reason I became extremely sad and depressed. After feeling sorry for myself for a while it became clear that something was wrong in this place. I quickly did a thorough room-cleansing and within a few minutes my mood changed completely and I once again felt happy and light.

Talking with the innkeeper later I learned that a friend of his who had lost his family in a terrible car accident had stayed in that room for some weeks before I arrived. I had apparently picked up the poor man's grief which was still clinging to the aura of the room. The Reiki room-cleansing cleared the heavy energies immediately.

Room—Cleansing with the Power Symbol

Prerequisite:

2nd Reiki Degree

Technical Instructions

Step 1: Stand relaxed with your feet parallel to each other in a corner of the space to be cleansed and take several deep breaths.

Step 2: Now draw the power symbol as large as possible with your hand once in one corner and mentally repeat the corresponding Mantra three times.

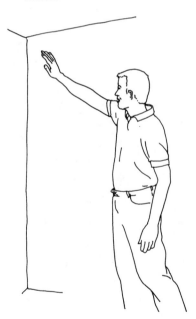

Draw the power symbol as large as possible in every corner of the room

Step 3: Either during or after saying the Mantra three times press the power symbol into the corner with both hands without touching the walls.

Step 4: Repeat the first three steps in every corner of the room.

I do this technique in the following way: I raise my left arm above my head and face the open hand towards the corner. While I do this I leave my right arm hanging next to my right thigh with its open hand also facing towards the corner. Then I push the power symbol three times respectively into the corner of the room. I treat the other three corners of the room the same way.

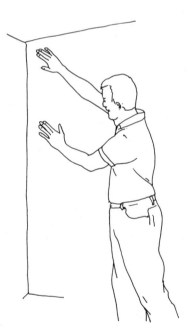

Now push the power symbol into all the corners of the room

Repeat this technique if you feel that the effect may have weakened but a one-time treatment is normally enough.

Length	Depends upon the size of the room. For example a hotel room needs 3 to 4 minutes.
Please Note	If there are people present who are not Reiki initiates draw the symbol mentally and project it with your eyes or forehead chakra into all four corners of the room.
Use	This technique helps to rid rooms and entire houses of vibrations that are unpleasant for you. If you travel a lot experiment with this in your next hotel room. If you work in a hospital cleanse the hospital rooms each time a patient is released or has died.
Combination	Grounding with the power symbol (see page 161).
Philosophy	Negative energies are not actually 'negative'. They simply vibrate at a frequency that is not compatible with your own. Reiki is compatible with all living beings. This is why you don't have to hesitate in treating any type of housing or place with Reiki. It works like the reset button in a speedometer. You can use it to reset the energy of any place back to its natural vibration. In the course of time it will naturally be imbued with the personal energy of the individual who lives there.

What Works? What Doesn't?

This technique can cleanse a room or a house. If however the disruptive factor returns, the old problem will probably arise again. If a room or house is haunted I suggest first calling the 'spirit' with the Reiki symbols of the 2nd Degree and asking it to stop its mischief. Spirits can be an embodiment of our own thoughts which through constant repetition have taken on a life of their own. They can also be the energetic remains of a person who has died there very suddenly. In this type of work it is important not to be afraid and always remember who is in charge here: the living!

Experiences   Unfortunately I currently spend more time in hotel rooms than at home. I use this technique whenever something inside me feels uncomfortable as I enter a room. This way I can sleep well wherever I am.

Safety on the Street with Reiki

Prerequisite:

2nd Reiki Degree

Technical Instructions

This technique has two phases. The first one protects us and the second one protects our vehicle be it a bicycle, a car or an airplane.

The 1st Phase:

Step 1: Sit down comfortably and take a few deep breaths.

Step 2: Draw the distance-treatment symbol once and mentally repeat the corresponding Mantra three times.

Step 3: Now repeat your name and the situation to be treated such as your drive to work, to the city or your vacation. Say: "For the length of this journey please let the Reiki force flow so that there will be harmony and safety for everyone involved."

Step 4: Draw the mental-healing symbol once and repeat the Mantra mentally three times.

Step 5: Stabilize everything with the power symbol (draw it once repeat the Mantra three times).

Step 6: Let the energy flow ....

The 2ⁿᵈ Phase: (On the Bicycle, In the Car, On the Plane)

Step 1: Sit down comfortably and draw the distance-treatment symbol once.

Step 2: Repeat the Mantra three times.

Step 3: Now repeat the description of the situation to be treated three times.

Step 4: Draw the mental-healing symbol once, repeat the Mantra three times and wrap your vehicle in it.

Step 5: Now draw the power symbol once, repeat the Mantra three times and send it to the front, back and sides of the vehicle.
In the car send it to both of the bumpers, on the plane to the engines and the wings, on a bicycle to both wheels, the handlebar and the chain. In the car you can also safeguard all of the mirrors with the power symbol.

Step 6: Let the energy flow ....
It can also be done by imagining holding the vehicle between your folded hands.

Length   2 to 5 minutes.

Please Note   It has been discovered that this technique seems to work better if you use it *before* the beginning of a journey.

Use   It can be used in traffic to protect you and others on the road.

Combination   Distant healing treatment for situations in the future, affirmation technique, grounding technique.

Philosophy People have known about positive energy fields for thousands of years. Every power spot has such a field of either natural or mystic origin. We can create power fields like these with Reiki. This is not a manipulation of our surroundings but rather an offering of harmony and love. Whether the other people on the road accept the offer is up to them. But deep down we humans all long for this and will accept it with gratitude.

What Works? What Doesn't?

There are two ways this technique can help in traffic: On the one hand it builds an energetic wall of protection. On the other it gives us self-assurance. We ourselves also have to take care. Reiki does not protect us from our own recklessness!

Experiences A Reiki friend has used this technique for years before she drives off in the car even if it is just to the corner supermarket. For her, driving a car is a necessary evil and with the help of this technique she has gained a great deal of confidence and a feeling of safety in traffic.

269

Sex with Reiki

Prerequisite:
2nd Reiki Degree

Technical Instructions

Before you go to bed with your partner or when you are already in bed together draw the distance-treatment symbol once, repeat the corresponding Mantra and both of your names three times. Send Reiki to both of you and to the bedroom or wherever you may be for the length of your time together. Then draw the mental-healing symbol once, repeat the Mantra three times and enclose both of you in a pyramid of harmony. Seal everything with the power symbol. You will have to figure out the rest on your own!

For men: If you have not been with a woman for a long time or suffer from premature ejaculation draw the power symbol mentally and send it to the root of the penis.

Length	Good question!
Please Note	Reiki does not help with birth control!
Use	This technique can be used for more joy and harmony during sex.
Combination	Distant healing treatment of a situation in the future, whole-body treatment, chakra treatment.
Philosophy	It is helpful when partners relate to life with similar levels of sensitivity. With this technique two

people can connect in the most intimate way and turn off, at least temporarily, the duality of individual existence.

The special technique for men is based on the fact that premature ejaculation is a widespread but treatable condition. Reiki brings us back to our natural state of existence, and this state is relaxed and happy!

What Works? What Doesn't?

Sexual problems are usually not related to the physical body and should be treated by a loving experienced therapist. Experience has shown that it is better not to discuss these problems with friends because the partner could easily feel betrayed. In any case it should first be talked about together.

This technique is especially helpful for inexperienced partners and those who are relatively unfamiliar with each other and their own bodies.

Experiences A married couple I know has practiced this technique since they were both initiated into 2nd Reiki Degree. They have said many times that their bedroom has now become a temple. A picture of the Amida Buddha now hangs there.

Systematic Chakra Work with Rainbow Reiki

Prerequisite:

1ˢᵗ Reiki Degree

Technical Instructions

Test Phase:

> With the help of the kinesiology arm tests (see the description on page 58) we can identify a weak chakra in relation to a specific issue. To do this the client thinks of the problem while the six major chakras are tested one by one.
>
> To test the chakras the testing hand is always held about one to two handwidths away from the chakra in question, palm facing it. A weakness in the test arm shows a momentary deficient functioning of the corresponding energy center relative to the problem.
>
> Once it is determined which chakra or chakras are weak we can begin with the treatment.

Application Phase:

> For a few minutes allow Reiki to be absorbed at a distance of one to two handwidths to the front and back of the body. In order to strengthen the flow of energy as you do so move your hands slightly. This is called the 'cloud hands' technique.

While receiving Reiki the client continues to think about the problem addressed in the test phase so that Reiki is directly drawn to the areas of the energy centers that are connected to the problem.

Finally the weak chakras should be tested one more time as described above to determine if the treatment has been a success. If a chakra isn't completely strong yet continue the treatment.

Length

The treatment for each chakra should last at least 3 minutes. If there are more serious difficulties it can also be extended to 5 to 10 minutes.

Please Note

A single treatment session is not necessarily enough for lasting harmonization of a problem. It is advisable to have a session two to three times a week until the symptoms have disappeared. The human body needs some time to integrate healing stimuli. Consequently treatments involving systematic chakra work more than once a day are normally only recommended in acute cases.

Use

The systematic chakra work can be used for virtually any problem. This includes the physical, emotional and mental levels.

Combination

Depending on the situation additional methods such as the whole-body treatment, special positions, intuitive Reiki, mental healing, Karma-Clearing or chakra balancing may be applied.

The systematic chakra work can also be used in a Reiki distant healing treatment. Only the arm test has to be done directly. Once these results have been obtained the treatment can begin.

273

Philosophy   The six major chakras represent and organize all of the important life themes, organs and body functions. If the major chakras are specifically harmonized and strengthened the ability to heal any problem is improved and healing processes often actually begin at this point. In accordance with the esoteric law: 'Energy flows where attention goes!', Reiki is specifically drawn to a chakra directly connected with the disharmony arising when the client thinks of the problem.

What Works? What Doesn't?

Systematic chakra work can very effectively contribute to harmonizing practically every type of imbalance. The success of the treatment however is limited by blocks that prevent the exchange of information between the treated chakras and the afflicted areas. This is why additional techniques need to be used to dissolve such blocks and generally improve the condition of the body.

Experiences   In my experience when helping smokers give up their habit the systematic chakra work makes a very constructive contribution to a speedy and lasting healing. I have very often been struck by how much more effective autosuggestion and healing-stone work are for this problem in conjunction with systematic chakra work.

Tantric Meditation with Rainbow Reiki

Prerequisite:

1st Reiki Degree

Technical Instructions

Step 1: The partners sit opposite and facing one another on the floor. Hold the palms of your hands so that they touch each other, i.e. the left hand of the one person on the right hand of the other and vice versa. Bend your legs and spread them at an angle of about 45°.

Step 2: Coordinate the breath so that both of you are breathing in the same rhythm. The breath should be directed in such a way that it alter-

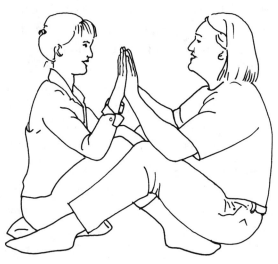

Enjoying togetherness in a new way with the Tantric meditation

nates between the hara, the energetic center just below the navel, and the 2nd chakra.

Step 3: Feel the energy flowing within you and between you!

Length 15 minutes or longer.

Please Note In addition build Reiki showers above each of you and draw power symbols on the palms of your hands. When strong feelings arise be sure to keep breathing into the *hara.*

Use Constructive support for the partnership, strengthening the quality of life and sensuality, deep emotional understanding, developing the ability to perceive energy.

Combination Reiki for the Inner Child, Reiki for the Higher Self of the partnership, mutual (alternating) whole-body treatment.

Philosophy By connecting the flow of energy of the partners through placing their palms on each other and synchronizing their breath, feelings become attuned and a pleasant loving exchange takes place. This creates more closeness, understanding and resonance. Practicing regularly each week, or daily during times of crisis, is the recipe for a lasting, stable deepening of the relationship.

What Works? What Doesn't?

With this exercise it is often astoundingly simple to create understanding and openness as well as a warm loving atmosphere. This does take time so it a good idea to spend more than 30 minutes on at least the first three sessions. Of course two people must talk together in order to clear up any conflicts that may arise and such discussions are much more constructive when the partners have meditated together beforehand. There needs to be a willingness to be conciliatory, to be truthful, to change and to be tolerant if the partnership is to work. It is also possible to heal deep crises when the opportunities provided by the Tantric partner meditation are used.

Experiences Some years ago a somewhat exotic experience with the partner meditation helped a couple I was working with to overcome a difficult situation Because the husband was sent to work in another country for a year leaving his wife and children at home, the whole family experienced a lot of fear, frustration and tension. Both of them had learned the 1st and 2nd Degree of Rainbow Reiki with me so I showed them how to meet together on a spiritual level using the distance-treatment technique and the partner meditation. They were enthusiastic about it and followed the technique together every evening for 15 minutes before going to sleep. Within a few days they both felt the return of harmony and were again full of love and trust for each other.

When the husband returned many months later, they both wrote me a letter saying that thanks to the partner meditation the time of separation helped them to understand their relationship in a completely new light and supported the intensification of their love for each other.

Throughout the Day—Giving Reiki

Prerequisite:

2nd Reiki Degree

Technical Instructions

Step 1: Draw the distance-treatment symbol once and repeat the Mantra three times mentally.*

Step 2: Say: "With the help of the Reiki symbols I am giving energy to the whole day."

Step 3: Now draw the mental-healing symbol once and repeat the Mantra three times.

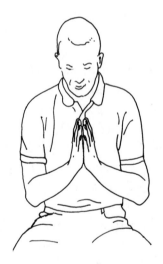

With the help of the Reiki symbols ...

---

* If you are working with a client say their name three times.

Step 4: Seal everything with the power symbol (draw it once and say the Mantra three times).

Step 5: Let the energy flow ....

Length 2 to 10 minutes.

Please Note This technique should, like all techniques of the distant healing treatment, only be practiced with the express permission of the recipient.

Use This technique can help us in providing the whole day and ourselves, since we are living this day, with fresh Reiki energy.

Combination Distant healing treatment, distant healing treatment of situations in the future.

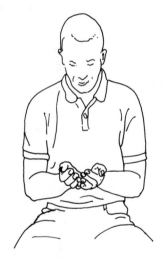

I am giving energy to the whole day

Philosophy   We have to drag our egos around with us all day long. But this has its up side in the continuing opportunity to be a witness to our programmed selves. This technique gives us the strength to do this and it is the only alchemy. Transformation comes only through dispassionate and detailed watching of the self moment by moment, all day long. The work we do on ourselves is the only thing that makes life worth living.

We arise from the source of all living beings. It is here that we have common ground with everything manifested in the natural world.

What Works? What Doesn't?

This technique will not make every wish come true. Reiki would not even be doing us a favor if it did. It is much more important to live with what we have, not constantly running after some dream or another, missing out on the only moment that we can actually experience: this moment, Here and Now.

Experiences   One of my students told me: "When I give Reiki to the whole day everything somehow runs like clockwork. I leave the house and the bus comes immediately. I don't have to wait for the subway and in the department store where I work the elevator always comes right after I press the button. If I don't send Reiki to the whole day I have to stand around until I'm ready to drop ...."

Whole-Body Protection with the Power Symbol

Prerequisite:

2nd Reiki Degree

Technical Instructions

Step 1: Stand in a relaxed way with both feet parallel to each other and take several deep breaths.

Step 2: Draw the power symbol once in the way that is most comfortable for you and repeat the Mantra three times mentally.

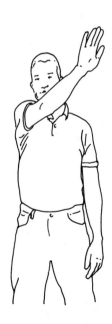 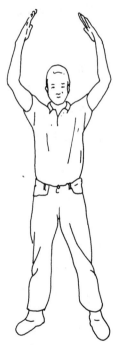

Draw the power symbol ...   *And wrap yourself in it*

Step 3: Now bring both hands together above your head with the palms facing you and slowly, like a window shutter closing let them move down along your entire body to the ground.

Step 4: Draw the power symbol once again and repeat the Mantra three times. Let an energy window shutter move down the back of you.

Step 5: Repeat this movement once each on your left and right side. The order doesn't matter.

Length   1 to 3 minutes.

Please Note   If you often feel vulnerable, 'too open' or threatened by psychic attacks you need learn how to transform negative energies. Walter teaches this throughout the world in special seminars.

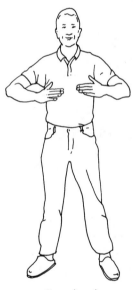

From head

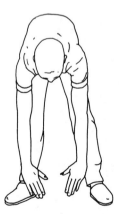

to foot

Use	This technique can be used whenever you want to protect yourself against something or someone.
Combination	Grounding technique (see page 161), Room cleansing with Rainbow Reiki (see page 259), Mental Healing with Rainbow Reiki (see page 209).
Philosophy	Our aura is our energetic protection shield. Just as a protective shield preserved the knights of old from injury, an intact aura defends and strengthens us.

What Works? What Doesn't?

This technique helps us to 'condense' our aura and as a result generates more self-confidence. If this is lacking in our basic nature we should also resort to other techniques that can help us develop this quality.

Experiences   A friend of mine who was a professional boxer for many years has spared himself lots of physical and mental injury with the help of this technique. It is also helpful in daily life until you have learned to completely open up instead of protecting yourself. However don't try this one out in the ring without prior training!

Working with Reiki

Prerequisite:

1st Reiki Degree

Technical Instructions

Step 1: Connect with the Reiki energy.

Step 2: Let the Reiki energy consciously flow during your work.

With a little bit of imagination this is possible in almost every situation you can imagine in every-

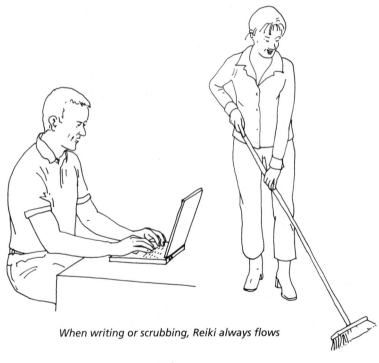

When writing or scrubbing, Reiki always flows

day life. Experiment in your own area. The possibilities are endless. Here are a few examples: When you play piano let the energy bubble out of your hands, your eyes and your heart in the direction of the piano and your listeners.

If you are working on a piece of furniture lovingly touch the material and let the energy flow into the process.

Hold your hammer with consciousness and the Reiki force!

Let the Reiki energy flow while you teach math in the classroom.

If you have received the 2nd Reiki Degree you can let the Reiki symbols flow into your work. For example, I always cook with the power symbol. If I use soy sauce I draw the power symbol on the food with it.

Length   As long as you like whenever you think of it. For example right now, this moment as you hold this book in your hands.

Please Note   If this technique distracts you when you are working don't use it while in traffic or during other risky types of work that call for full concentration until you have more practice with it. You can practice using it while reading, walking or doing the dishes. But be careful with the Meissener porcelain!

Use   This technique can be used to let Reiki flow into your daily work.

Combination   Distant healing treatment, Objects—Treatment with Reiki, treatment of future situations.

Philosophy   Reiki not only has a healing effect on the body and mind. It also enriches all of our actions improving the quality of life. Over the course of time this technique can help us feel our best in any situation. I have noticed that my personal weaknesses often become less important when I work in this manner.

What Works? What Doesn't?

The end results of any type of work can virtually never be predicted. Even if we are praised and paid well for doing the work it really doesn't mean much. It can also go the other way. The important thing is how we feel about it and how we feel about ourselves. I work according to the following principle: 'Do your best and don't expect anything'. This can also protect us from disappointments.

Experiences   For many years now I have used Reiki while I write. I hope that this shows through!

Appendix

Also by Walter Lübeck:

The Complete Reiki Handbook, Lotus Press.

Introduction to the Reiki practice, whole-body and chakra treatments, the ABCs of the special positions, Reiki meditation, Reiki and healing stones, the theory of chakras and much more.

Reiki—Way of the Heart, Lotus Press.

The Reiki story, precise descriptions of the individual Reiki Degrees, Rainbow Reiki resonance therapy, psychological theory of chakras.

Reiki for First Aid, Lotus Press.

More than 40 different whole-body treatments specifically for individual health disorders. With herbal and nutritional naturopathy.

Rainbow Reiki, Lotus Press.

Introduction to the fundamentals of Rainbow Reiki, crystal mandalas, Reiki Essences, work with angels and power spots, and much more.

The Spirit of Reiki, Lübeck/Petter/Rand, Lotus Press.

The topics presented in a uniquely condensed form in this book range from the tradition to the present: fundamental lines of transmission, original writings, mastery, symbols, techniques, treatments and Reiki as a spiritual path in life .... This is the book for Reiki experts who enjoy learning new things and having an overview of the international developments in the Reiki streams.

The Chakra Energy Cards, Lotus Press.

This extensive card set is suitable for all forms of energy healing and Reiki treatments.

The special characteristic of this new edition is the healing symbols of the Great Goddess and her angels. The card set contains healing affirmations as well as a healing symbol for each area in the subtle energy centers of the major and secondary chakras as well as the auric fields. It invites us to take a playful and creative approach in dealing with the powers of the energy bodies—and also supports all types of healing work. Although the Chakra Energy Cards are a complete method by themselves they can also be integrated into almost any other spiritual system.

Pendulum Healing Handbook, Lotus Press.

Based on years of seminar practice this book provides precise instructions for the correct way to use a pendulum, the best way to work with pendulum tables and important tips for advanced practitioners. It gives a detailed explanation of how the ability to use a pendulum can be awakened and developed even if 'nothing is moving'. Includes a comprehensive collection of pendulum tables.

Aura Healing Handbook, Lotus Press.

An instruction manual for reading auras and chakras which as a standard work has been used by many professionals throughout the world. It contains detailed, precise descriptions of the subtle energy system, the major and secondary chakras, the auric field, the muscle-armor rings and the energy organs. Also explains how to read the chakras with the *I Ching,* the Chinese Book of Changes.

The Tao of Money, Lotus Press.

About the spiritual approach to money, profession (calling) and possessions. How holistic wealth is created and meaningfully used for the good of the whole.

L-Carnitine, Lotus Press.

An extensive book on what is probably the best-researched nutritional supplement in the world, using L-carnitine for healthy weight-loss, fit and healthy in old age, pregnancy and children, leisure sports, increasing and stabilizing physical and psychological performance, healing effects for various health problems.

Healing Power of Pau D'Arco, Lotus Press.

A book about one of the most effective medicinal plants in the world, scientific studies, reports on experiences, ethno medicine, the best recipes.

Also by Frank Arjava Petter:

Reiki Fire, Lotus Press.

An absolutely practical Reiki guide. The heart, the body, the mind and the esoteric background—this book covers it all. In addition it is a good introduction to the background of Reiki as it is still taught and lived today in Japan.

Reiki—The Legacy of Dr. Usui, Lotus Press.

The publication of the rediscovered documents on the origins and developments of the Reiki system as well as new aspects of Reiki energy.

The Original Reiki Handbook of Dr. Usui, Lotus Press.

The classic work of Reiki. The original system as taught by Dr. Mikao Usui. This is a revised version of the textbook that

Dr. Mikao Usui gave to his students—illustrated with many color photos of the exact treatment instructions.

The Spirit of Reiki, Lübeck/Petter/Rand, Lotus Press.

→ A description of this book can be found under books by Walter Lübeck.

The Hayashi Reiki Manual, Petter/Yamaguchi/Hayashi, Lotus Press.

The story of Dr. Chujiro Hayashi, the highly renowned student of Reiki founder, Dr. Mikao Usui, newly researched and sensationally illustrated with previously unpublished archive photos. The manual includes Reiki techniques never taught in the West before as well as specific documents such as the original certificates of Dr. Hayashi.

About the Authors

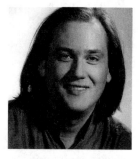

Walter Lübeck

Walter Lübeck (Aquarius, Asc. Sagittarius) has been active as a spiritual teacher since 1988. He teaches his own Rainbow Reiki System, Three-Rays Meditation and Lemurian Tantra in both English and German throughout the world. The three principles of personal responsibility, love and consciousness are an important guideline for him in his private and professional life. With his work he seeks to contribute to the earliest possible dawning of a new Golden Age on Earth.

Walter has made the results of his research available to the public in his 20 books (7 of which are on Reiki). These have been translated into more than a dozen languages. He has also published diverse articles in specialized magazines and teaching videos.

It is very important, he finds, for spiritual knowledge to be used to increase the holistic quality of life. With his diversified training in Reiki, meditation, NLP, shamanism, tantra, homeopathy, nutrition, inner martial arts, Feng Shui and work with crystals he attempts to unite the various esoteric paths and their knowledge. He seeks to give optimal help to his students as they progress on their individual paths.

An enthusiastic musician Walter likes to use drums, didgeridoo, voice and dance in rituals and spiritual healing. He is a recording artist (CD *Rainbow Trance)*.

Contact: www.rainbowreiki.net

Frank Arjava Petter

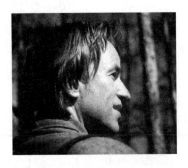

In 1993 Frank Arjava Petter brought Reiki from the West back to the land of its origin and was the first European to teach the Reiki Master/Teacher Degree in Japan. In the subsequent years he followed the various branches of Reiki to their roots in the original Reiki of Dr. Mikao Usui and Dr. Chujiro Hayashi. Along with many exciting historical facts he discovered fascinating healing techniques sourced from the beginnings of this wonderful system.

Frank Arjava Petter currently teaches original Reiki techniques worldwide in lectures and seminars. His books *Reiki Fire, Reiki—The Legacy of Dr. Usui, The Original Reiki Handbook of Dr. Mikao Usui* and *The Hayashi Reiki Manual* have already become international bestsellers. He also gives seminars and offers advanced trainings in Bert Hellinger's Family Constellations, as well as courses in meditation and the art of living in the present.

Contact: www.ReikiDharma.com

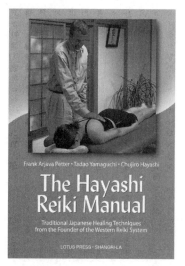

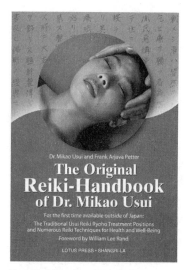

Frank Arjava Petter · Tadao Yamaguchi
Chujiro Hayashi

The Hayashi Reiki Manual

Traditional Japanese Healing Techniques from the Founder of the Western Reiki System

Dr. Chujiro Hayashi is the highly renowned student of Reiki founder, Dr. Mikao Usui. Dr. Hayashi developed his own style of Reiki and became the teacher of Hawayo Takata, who introduced Reiki to the West.

However, Dr. Hayashi also taught Reiki to Japanese students such as young Chiyoko Yamaguchi, born in 1920. She is still practicing today—and Frank Arjava Petter was allowed to become her student and learn the original Hayashi Reiki system from her.

The manual presents the story of Dr. Hayashi, newly researched and sensationally illustrated with previously unpublished archive photos, Reiki techniques never taught in the West before, and specific documents such as the original certificates of Dr. Hayashi.

full color ·112 pages · $19.95
ISBN 0-914955-75-6

Dr. Mikao Usui and Frank A. Petter

The Original Reiki Handbook of Dr. Mikao Usui

The Traditional Usui Reiki Ryoho Treatment Positions and Numerous Reiki Techniques for Health and Well-Being

For the first time available outside of Japan: The original hand positions from Dr. Usui's handbook, illustrated with 100 colored photos.

The hand positions for a great variety of health complaints have been listed in detail, making it a valuable reference work for anyone who practices Reiki.

Now, that the original handbook has been translated into English, Dr. Usui's hand positions and healing techniques can be studied directly for the first time. Whether you are an initiate or a master, if you practice Reiki you can expand your knowledge dramatically as you follow in the footsteps of a great healer.

100 photos · 80 pages · $14.95
ISBN 0-914955-57-8

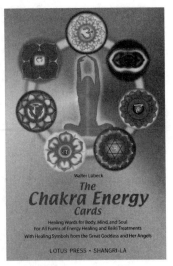

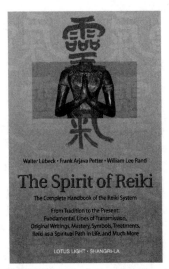

Walter Lübeck

The Chakra Energy Cards

Healing Words for Body, Mind, and Soul

For All Forms of Energy Healing and Reiki Treatments

With Healing Symbols from the Great Goddess and Her Angels

Each card has a special healing symbol, which conveys its message directly to the user. The cards spark gentle processes of healing and inspire us in a loving way. Supplemented in the accompanying handbook by helpful suggestions for actions that offer support in resolving and releasing stuck energies. *The Chakra Energy Cards* offer a complete method by themselves, yet they can also be integrated into almost any other spiritual system, especially Reiki. The effect of each card can be optimally complemented with the specific use of the healing gemstones, fragrance essences, and Bach Flowers.

Set (book and card pack) with 192-page handbook and 154 Chakra Energy Cards · $24.95
ISBN 0-914955-72-1

W. Lübeck / F.A. Petter / W.L. Rand

The Spirit of Reiki

The Complete Handbook of the Reiki System

From Tradition to the Present: Fundamental, Lines of Transmission, Original Writings, Mastery, Symbols, Treatments, Reiki as a Spiritual Path in Life, and Much More

Never before, have three Reiki masters from different lineages and with such extensive background come together to share their experience.

A wealth of information on Reiki never before brought together in one place. The broad spectrum of topics range from the search for a scientific explanation of Reiki energy to Reiki as a spiritual path. It also includes the latest understanding of Dr. Usui's original healing methods, how Reiki is currently practiced in Japan, an analysis of the Western evolution of Reiki, and a discussion about the direction Reiki is likely to take in the future.

150 photos and b/w illustrations
312 pages · $19.95
ISBN 0-914955-67-5

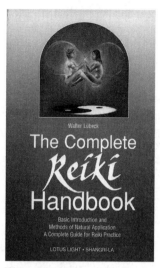

Walter Lübeck

The Complete Reiki Handbook

Basic Introduction and Methods of Natural Application—A Complete Guide for Reiki Practice

This is a complete guide for Reiki practice and a wonderful tool for the necessary adjustment to the changes inherent in a new age. The author's style of natural simplicity, much appreciated by the readers of his many bestselling books, wonderfully complements this basic method for accessing universal life energy. He shares with us, as only a Reiki master can, the personal experience accumulated in his years of practice. Lovely illustrations of the different positions make the information as easily accessible visually as the author's direct and undogmatic style of writing. This work also offers a synthesis of Reiki and many other popular forms of healing.

192 pages · $14.95
ISBN 0-941524-87-6

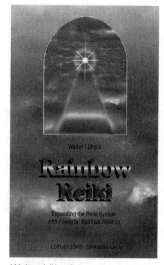

Walter Lübeck

Rainbow Reiki

Expanding the Reiki System with Powerful Spiritual Abilities

Rainbow Reiki gives us a wealth of possibilities to achieve completely new and different things with Reiki than taught in the traditional system. Walter Lübeck has tested these new methods in practical application for years and teaches them in his courses. Making Reiki Essences, performing guided aura and chakra work, connecting with existing power places and creating new personal ones, as well as developing Reiki Mandalas, are all a part of this system. This work is accompanied by plants devas, crystal teachers, angels of healing stones, and other beings of the spiritual world.

184 pages · $14.95
ISBN 0-914955-28-4

Herbs and other natural health products and information are often available at natural food stores or metaphysical bookstores. If you cannot find what you need locally, you can contact one of the following sources of supply.

Sources of Supply:

The following companies have an extensive selection of useful products and a long track-record of fulfillment. They have natural body care, aromatherapy, flower essences, crystals and tumbled stones, homeopathy, herbal products, vitamins and supplements, videos, books, audio tapes, candles, incense and bulk herbs, teas, massage tools and products and numerous alternative health items across a wide range of categories.

WHOLESALE:

Wholesale suppliers sell to stores and practitioners, not to individual consumers buying for their own personal use. Individual consumers should contact the RETAIL supplier listed below. Wholesale accounts should contact with business name, resale number or practitioner license in order to obtain a wholesale catalog and set up an account.

Lotus Light Natural Body Care
P. O. Box 1008
Silver Lake, WI 531 70 USA
800 548 3824 (toll free order line)
262 889 8501 (office phone)
website: www.lotuslight.com
email: lotuslight@lotuspress.com

RETAIL:

Retail suppliers provide products by mail order direct to consumers for their personal use. Stores or practitioners should contact the wholesale supplier listed above.

Internatural
P.O. Box 489
Twin Lakes, WI 53181 USA
800 643 4221 (toll free order line)
262 889 8581 (office phone)
email: internatural@internatural.com
website: www.internatural.com

Web site includes an extensive annotated catalog of more than 14,000 products that can be ordered "on line" for your convenience 24 hours a day, 7 days a week.